FEEL YOURSELF

FEEL YOURSELF

Ekbal Apol

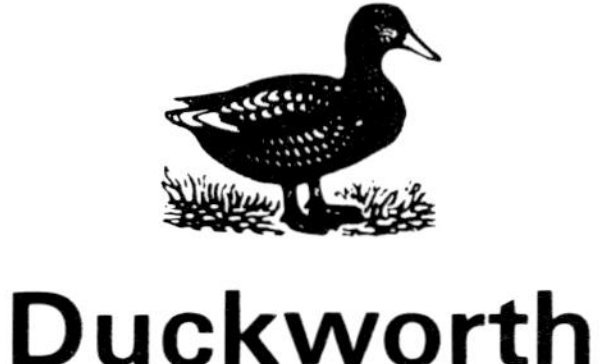

Duckworth

First published in 1979 by
Gerald Duckworth & Co. Ltd
The Old Piano Factory
43 Gloucester Crescent, London NW1

First published in USA 1979 by
Duckworth
4951 Top Line Drive
Dallas
Texas 75247

ISBN 0 7156 1147 X (Cased)
ISBN 0 7156 1148 8 (Paper)

Photoset in Great Britain by
Specialised Offset Services Limited, Liverpool
and printed by
Unwin Brothers Limited, Old Woking

CONTENTS

INTRODUCTION

In [mankind's] mighty limbs all things in Heaven and Earth are contained.
William Blake, *Jerusalem*

We human animals, unlike most other living beings, have come to rely less and less upon our bodies in our daily existence. Few of us have the opportunity to become aware of our bodies as total organisms. Even those whose work involves heavy manual labour are plagued with aches, pains, and lack of energy. Perhaps this last is due to overexertion and excessive use of specific parts of the organism at the expense of the whole. Entertainment is provided for us with a push of a button. Trains, planes, and cars move us from one place to another. Our bodies seem to be almost alien entities.

This book provides numerous exercises aimed at increasing physical self-awareness. We must relearn to use our bodies. Body and mind must act together in this effort. The body, of course, is constantly changing in response to such 'realities' as hereditary factors, conditioning, ageing, environment, diet. Yet, whether we live in a rural paradise or an urban metropolis, whether we eat steak or drink carrot juice, our basic home is inside. We remain in this home until the body's physical functions cease.

The body is an extremely sophisticated and interconnected organism. Nerves, muscles, blood vessels, bones, lymph vessels, and organs function together in close physical proximity and maintain a real state of interdependency. Dis-ease can easily spread from one point or area of the body to another. The opposite is also true: increased energy and awareness will spread throughout the body as a result of the various exercises and massages described in this book. Of necessity, the exercises have had to be grouped according to the major areas that they affect. However, many of the exercises could easily fit into several chapters. As you perform them and feel soreness in legs, neck, back, shoulders, or pelvis, you will realise how interconnected your insides actually are.

Physical awareness not only involves being able to stand on your head; it also means knowing without counting how many steps you have just climbed on the way up to a friend's fifth-floor flat. Since most of us have lost the ability to move naturally, re-contacting our bodies requires a concentrated effort. The unconscious movements of our bodies – those that we are not aware of – reveal a lot about the mind, heart, and physical condition of the whole person. If you have the desire to grow and expand your physical self-awareness with exercise and concentration, this desire will be reflected in your unconscious movements and your ability to communicate with yourself and others. This is a process; the only judge of its success is you.

And you will feel better, stronger, healthier – not only when doing these exercises, but whenever you move. Much of our day is spent in movements of various kinds. Brushing the hair, for example, combines scalp massage with neck and face movement. Feel your body as it reacts to and moves with the brush. All movement, no matter how common or how simple, is an expression of how we feel, how our bodies feel: picking up crumbs from the floor, washing hands, stretching for an object high up in a cabinet, walking, running for a bus, moving while in a bath tub, turning round in a car. Even while sitting you can exercise your wrists, spine, buttocks, legs, or work on breathing. Basically, express yourself and your energy whenever you move. It is good to change your movements so that patterns will not develop and rigidify. New movements keep the body flowing.

As you become more involved in and aware of your body, you will slowly overcome the resistance that has been created over the years. At first, especially in certain of the exercises, your body will rebel. You will feel pain as unused muscles stretch. Your body will try to tell you that it cannot do this. It is important to remember that awareness and growth are, in fact, painful processes. This is true on a physical as well as on emotional and spiritual levels. The transitions from infant to child to adolescent to adult are difficult. Yet there is a real difference between 'cannot' and 'will not'. A person may say that he or she cannot drive a car; but it is not a physical impossibility – only a matter of will, energy, and concentration. We try to face situations and problems as we encounter them. So it must be with our bodies. To use extreme examples, after death and during hypnosis the body can be moved and directed in ways that seem impossible in our 'ordinary' state. Yet these extraordinary conditions are real; in these states our resistance is overcome, our bodies are relaxed. In the process of self-awareness, we become able to control the resistance ourselves. What was impossible and painful becomes possible and satisfying.

Though this book begins at the beginning, there is no set order in which to proceed. If you feel strain in your neck, perhaps you can start there. Or perhaps you will choose an exercise at random. As breathing is so basic to this book, and to life, it would be useful first to read at least the introduction to Chapter 1. Each of us has our own individual corpus, so each of us will experience the effort in our own way at our own pace. The timing, duration, and sequence of the exercises are up to you. Suggestions have been included in the text; but these are only guidelines – not rules. Perhaps you will find it satisfying and invigorating to work on an exercise once a day or once a month. You may find it more interesting and enlivening to work through some of these exercises with a partner. The results should be at least as productive as if each of you had worked on them separately. Chapter 9 contains exercises that are especially structured for two people working together. However, there are many other exercises in the book that can be practised with a partner.

The exercises are put together in convenient sequences. But you can do just part of many exercises, or create your own using some of the movements in this book. The exercises have not been handed down by divine law. They are examples which can start you on the path to discovering the unique needs of your own body.

It is especially in self-massage that you will find tensions and energy blockages. The main pressure points of each part of the body are denoted in drawings in the introduction to each chapter. These points, as they are the foci for energy flow in each specific area, are very responsive to touch and massage. All the exercises in this book can be considered as self-massage. Chapter 8 describes one specific method of direct massage for the face and head. Chapter 2 presents an indirect approach through the pressure points of the feet and hands. Self-massage is a powerful example of the use of your own resources and energy to heal a dis-eased part of you. There is a real interconnection between the exercises, work on the pressure points, and self-massage. These three elements together will increase your energy and strengthen your body.

Although physical pain will be encountered, it is important at the same time to be relaxed. Repetition of an exercise in a relaxed state of mind can enable you to progress much further over a period of time. It is unnatural constantly to push your body. The instruction 'repeat many times' appears throughout this book. Although there is no rule as to the 'best' number of times to repeat an exercise, 25 is often considered a standard and enables you to build up a good amount of energy, change muscle tonus, and create a natural rhythm for the desired movement in unison with appropriate breathing. An interesting experiment in this regard is to choose a particular exercise, lie on your back on the floor, close your eyes, and imagine your body working through the steps of the exercise. Visualise and feel your body as it stretches, tilts, rotates, and returns 25 times. Co-ordinate your breathing with this imagined effort. Then perform the exercise using your arms, back, legs, or whatever. Is it easier or more familiar? The body and mind must work together.

So, put on some comfortable clothes, sit down, relax, take a few deep breaths, feel the life flowing in and out. *Feel yourself.*

1. BREATHING

The amount of air that can be expelled in the deepest possible expiration, after the deepest possible inspiration, is called the vital capacity. This is the exchangeable volume of the lungs. It is not the total volume of the lungs, for they contain about a litre and a half of air, which could be released only if the chest walls were cut open and air allowed to escape. The vital capacity should be in harmony with the body's weight and height. It can be measured by the time it takes to empty the lungs. A healthy person, taking in as much air as possible and then singing a note at the pitch of his speaking voice, can hold this note for about 20 seconds. The exercises in this chapter will strengthen your lungs and increase your vital capacity. The more air is inhaled, the bigger we can blow up the balloon. People who regularly practise sports, run, or sing usually have a good vital capacity.

If the vital capacity is insufficient, the whole organism will be affected. The cells of the body are in constant need of oxygen. By breathing fast and often the body replenishes cells and overcomes any lack of oxygen. Breathing is so basic an activity in our life that we are rarely conscious of it. This does not mean, however, that breathing is an independent function. In fact, breathing can be controlled voluntarily, at least within certain limits. There is a direct relationship between the speed of breathing and the rate of heartbeat. Slowly increasing inspiration of air increases the amount expired, slows the heartbeat, and delays the next inbreath. Likewise, the more vigorously and forcefully we move our bodies, the faster our heartbeat.

Unless otherwise indicated in the exercises, inhale and exhale through the nose.

On page 9 you will find some of the most common movements encountered in this book. They are divided into two groups: breathing in and breathing out. Breathe in during movements which naturally include expansion of the lungs. In transition from one movement to another, breathe in as you enter a comfortable position. Contrariwise, when entering a difficult position, breathe out. This will decrease tension by relaxing the mind and the body's resistance to effort or pain. Exhaling during a strenuous movement results in most economic use of energy, in addition to preparing the body for a subsequent deep inhalation to provide the maximum amount of oxygen for muscles to do their work. This concentrated action improves coordination, provides a relaxed framework to balance the physical exertion or strain of the movement, and increases the amount of energy available to you. An example of an incorrect reaction would be inhaling and holding the breath while receiving a tetanus shot or the like. This would only create further tension and resistance. Exhaling at the time of injection is far more soothing. When holding a position or experiencing some pain, relaxed deep breathing is the proper response. You may have to practise to regain the natural rhythm of breathing to enhance your ability to do the exercises and feel healthier. It is worth the effort.

WHEN TO BREATHE IN AND OUT

arching spine – in
assuming comfortable position – in
assuming difficult position – out
bending knee – out
raising arms – in
stretching up – in
bending down – out
transition from one position to next – out
bouncing – out
contracting stomach and chest muscles – out
stretching leg upward – out
experiencing pain – out
forward bend – out
intense stretch, pain – out
relaxing – out
twisting – out
swinging legs upward – out
assuming balance position – out
raising arms and legs – out
pushing up, physical exertion – out

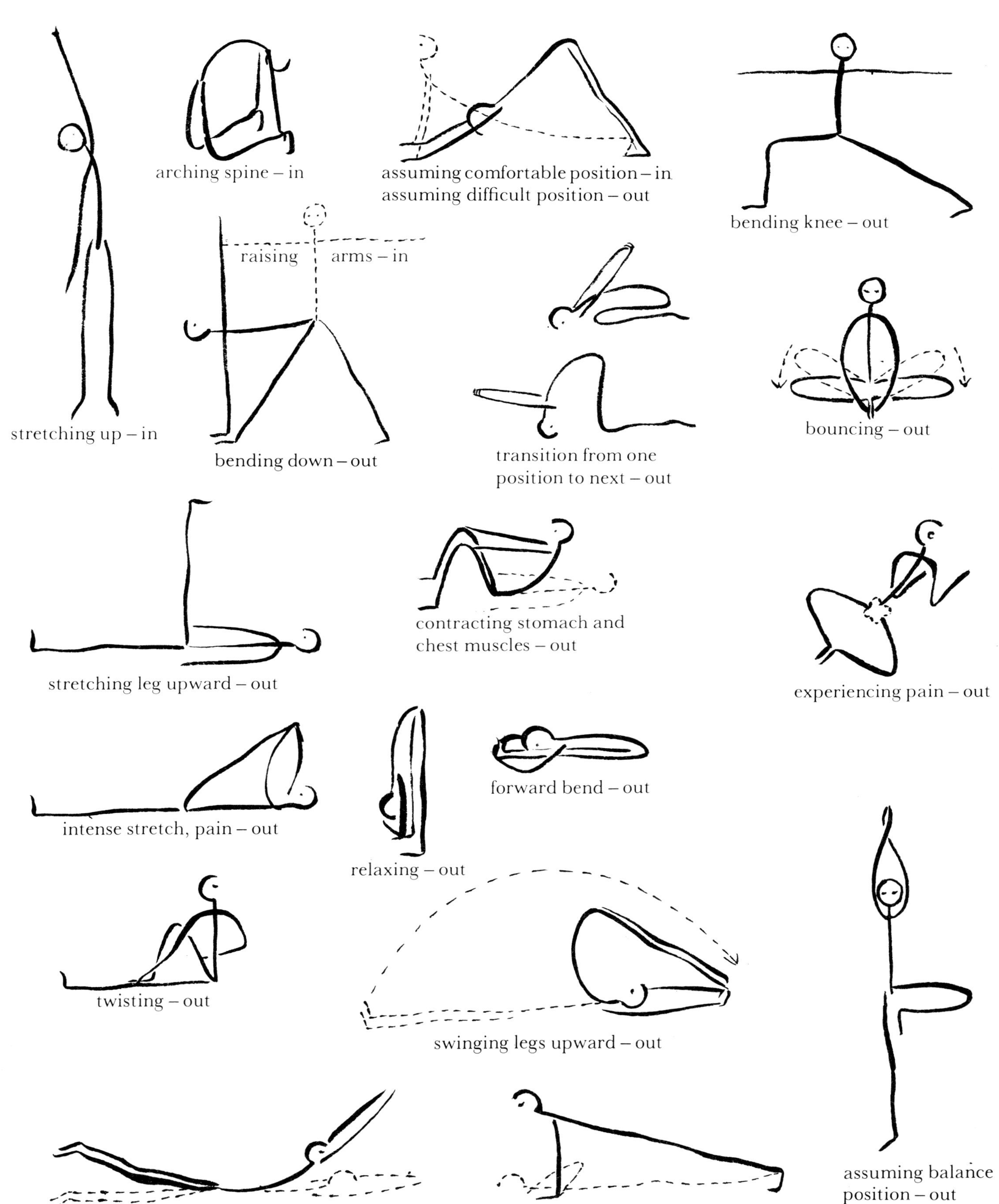

EXERCISE I:
THREE-PHASE BREATHING

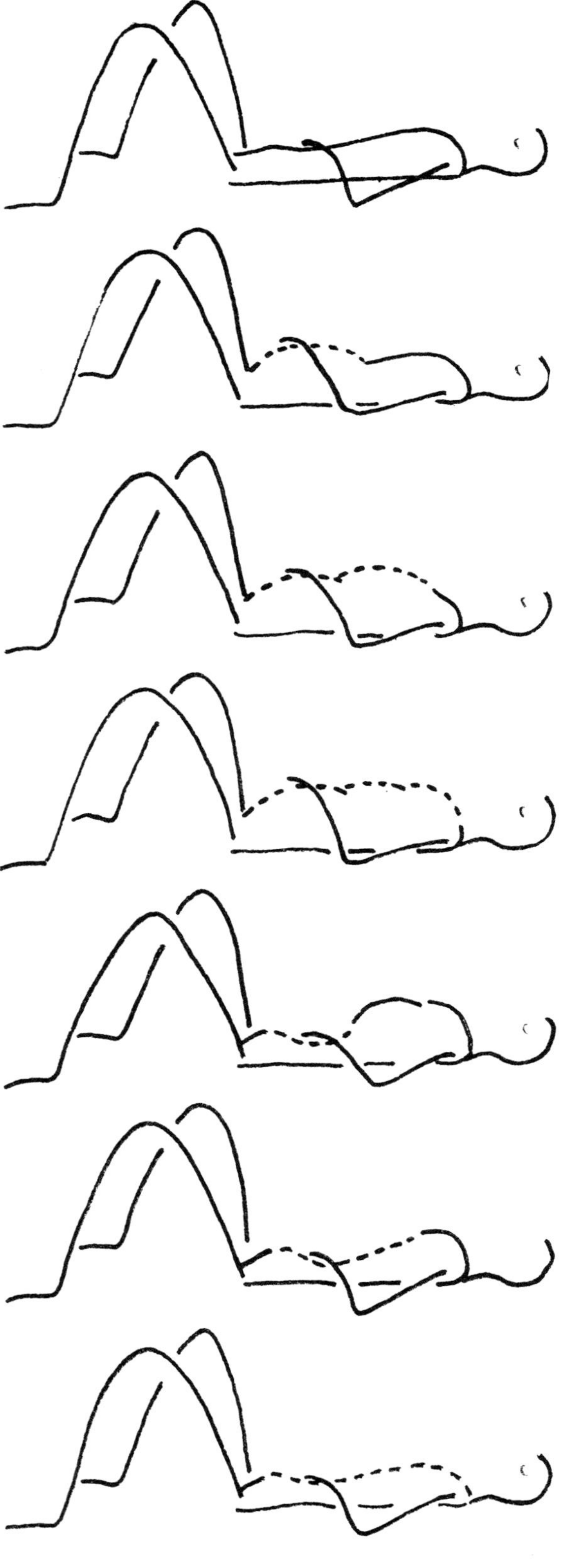

1. Lie down on your back. Relax. Rest both hands one on top of the other on stomach over the navel. Bring knees up, so that feet are one foot from buttocks.

2. Inhale through nose while pushing your hands upward with stomach muscles. Exhale. This first phase pulls down the diaphragm, a thick sheath separating lungs and heart from the abdomen, and allows the lower part of the lungs to expand. (See drawing p. 12.)

3. Repeat step 2. Then expand chest by raising chestbone upward and away from spine. Also expand chest sideways. Do not move back off floor. Exhale.

4. Inhale as in first two steps; then fill upper part of lungs under collarbone.

5. Now concentrate on breathing out. Exhale through the mouth, making a clear 'oo' sound at the pitch of your speaking voice. Move hands downward so as to push stomach in.

6. Then contract chest.

7. Finally empty upper part of chest (lungs). Repeat this three-stage breathing for about ten minutes without jerks or strain.

Continued performance will regulate blood pressure and improve the vital capacity. This exercise is comparable to yogic meditation practices in which the sound 'om' is constantly chanted. We use 'oo' here, as this sound produces the longest-lasting outbreath.

EXERCISE II

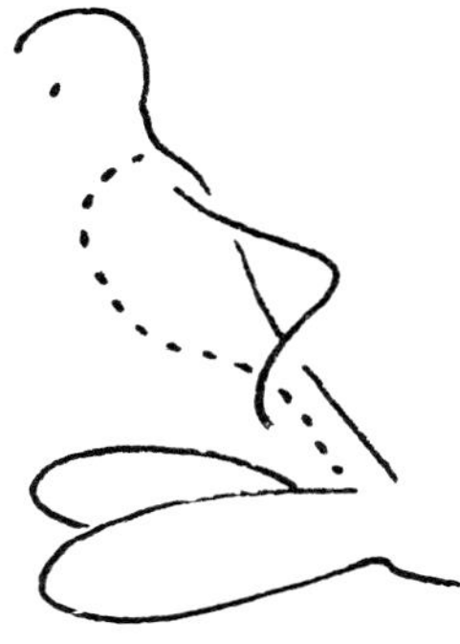

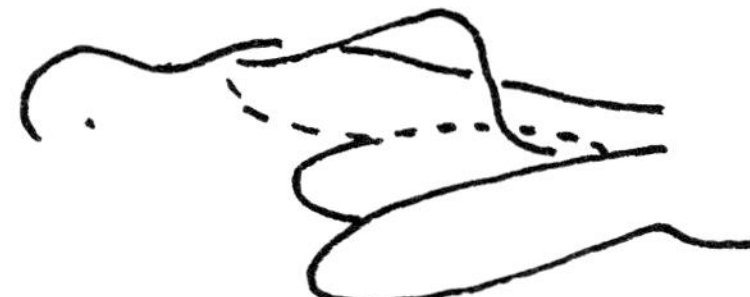

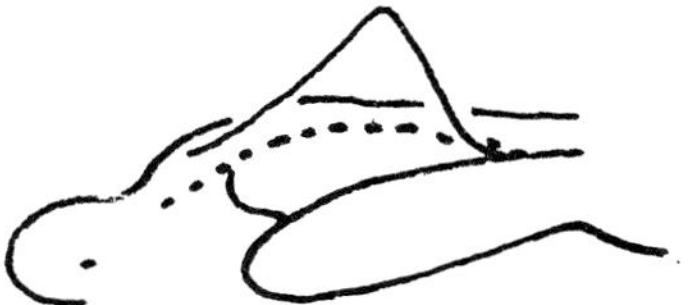

1. Sit in a comfortable position. Breathe in. Place both hands over the navel. Push stomach in against the spine and begin to exhale.
2. Continue exhaling, while contracting chest and bending forward from waist until chest touches thighs.
3. Exhalation is complete when forehead touches the floor.

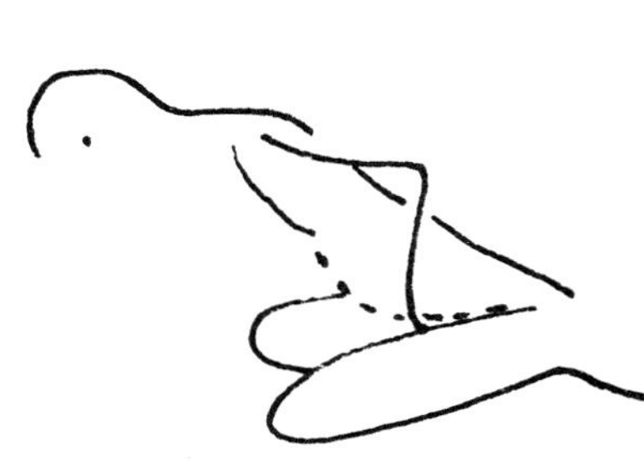

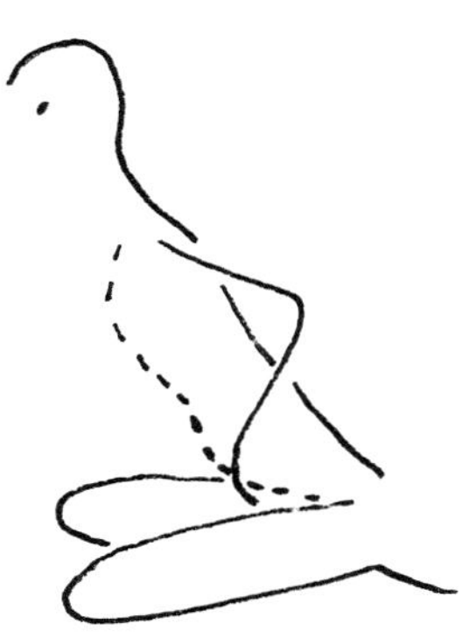

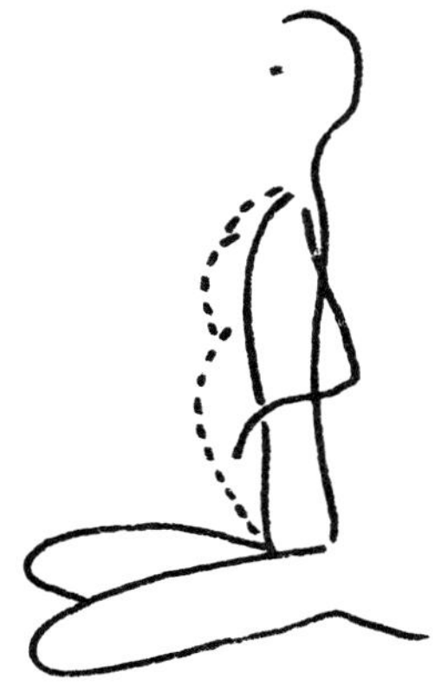

4. Pull up from waist, while slowly inhaling, so as to expand stomach; and push hands forward.
5. Continue inhaling, so as to expand chest; and move chestbone upward.
6. Finally, fill upper part of chest under collarbone. The inhalation should be complete when back is in an upright position.
7. Now exhale slowly, making a clear 'oo' sound, bending forward as illustrated and described in the first three steps. Inhale as in the last three steps. Repeat for ten minutes. As this exercise is more strenuous for the heart than the first, you may allow for half a minute's rest between each repetition.

The three-phase breathing exercises you have just done are good to practise after completing all other exercises, after a tiring day or before going to sleep. Both may also be performed silently, as it is sometimes inappropriate to 'oo' too loudly. For example, if you are suffering from insomnia and your partner is sleeping like a rose, you can do the breathing silently – if you have practised it aloud previously. Instead of uttering 'oo', simply whisper it, while directing your breath toward the ceiling. Ten minutes of concentrated effort will help you get to sleep.

EXERCISE III:
AWARENESS OF BREATHING

Lie down on back. Relax. Breathe softly and quietly. Close eyes.
Move awareness to the nostrils. Feel how the air flows in and out. Continue for one minute.
Now breathe in and follow air flow from your nostrils (1) to the upper part of the palate (2).
Then breathe out and follow the return of air from palate (2) to nostrils (1).
Continue for one minute.

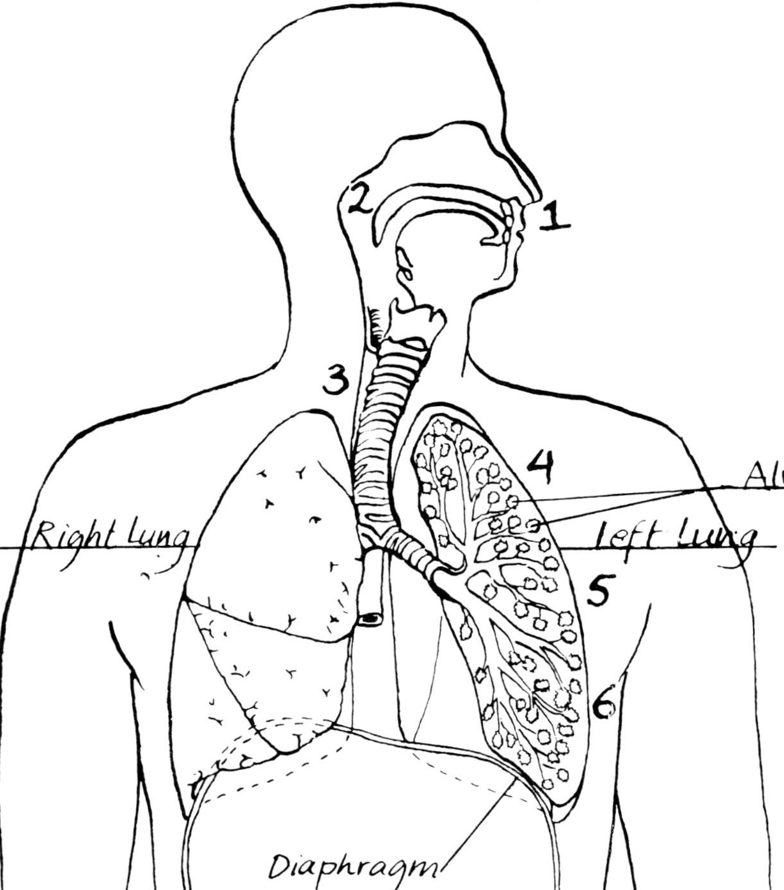

Again breathe in. Move your awareness from 1 to 2 to 3, the windpipe. Then breathe out from 3 to 2 to 1.
Continue for one minute.

Then breathe in, feeling flow from 1–2–3–4 upper part of the lungs. Breathe out from 4–3–2–1.
Continue for one minute.

Breathe in. The air flows from 1–2–3–4–5 middle part of lungs. Breathe out. Air flows from 5–4–3–2–1.
Continue for one minute.

Breathe in from 1–2–3–4–5–6 lower part of lungs.
Breathe out from 6–5–4–3–2–1.
Continue for one minute.

Continue from ten minutes to half an hour. This exercise is a process. The times given are not to be followed with the second-hand of a watch. It is important to feel the gradual movement of air-flow through the respiratory system. Some stages may take more time and concentration than others.

EXERCISE IV

Lie down on your back. Relax. Open your mouth and let the air escape quietly. Close mouth and move your throat as if you were swallowing something. Wait quietly for the next inbreath. Do not prevent the body from breathing in, but do not initiate the inbreath until the body does so by itself. When the inbreath comes, let the air flow in freely through the nose. Do not hold the breath. Exhale through the mouth and swallow. Wait. Gradually the waiting periods will last longer and longer.

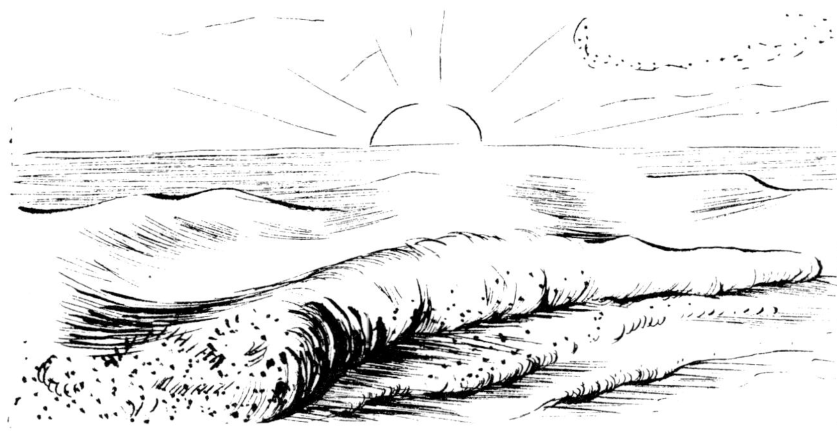

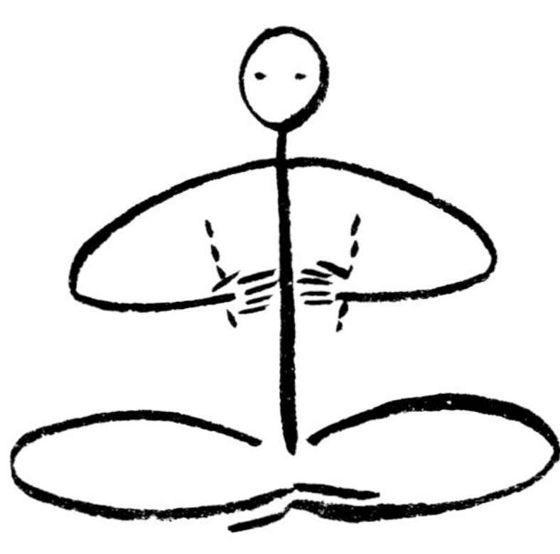

EXERCISE V

1. Sit either cross-legged or in the easy position: heel of one foot rests against the pubic bone; other foot rests comfortably in front of, and touching, first foot. Inhale deeply in three stages, as practised earlier. Hold. While holding breath, vigorously pat the front and side of chest with fast rhythmical movements.

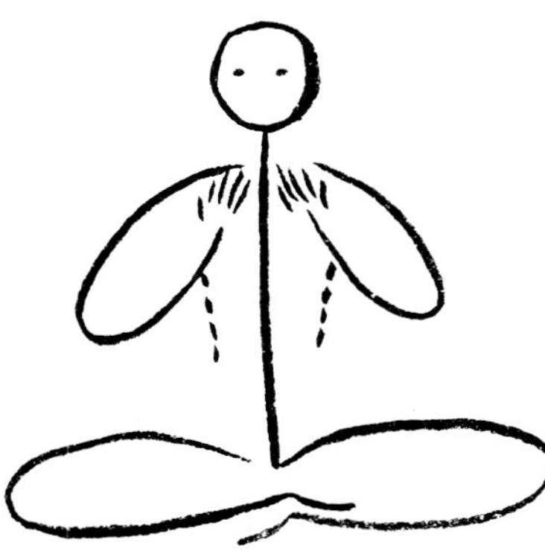

2. Then pat the upper part of the chest.

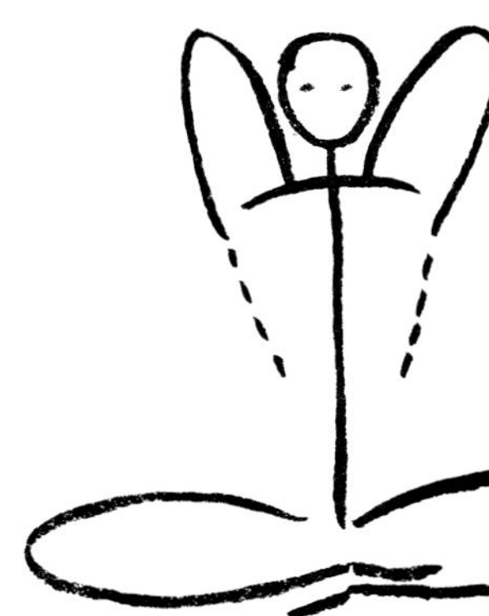

3. Then the upper part of the back, above the shoulder blades.

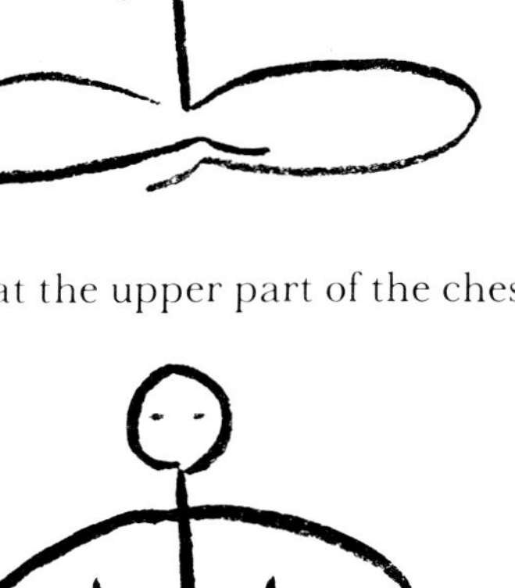

4. Then the back of the ribs, using the back of the hands.

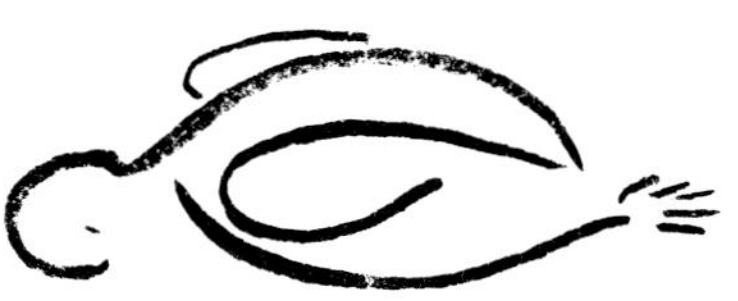

5. Bend forward and exhale fully. Repeat entire exercise at least three times.

EXERCISE VI

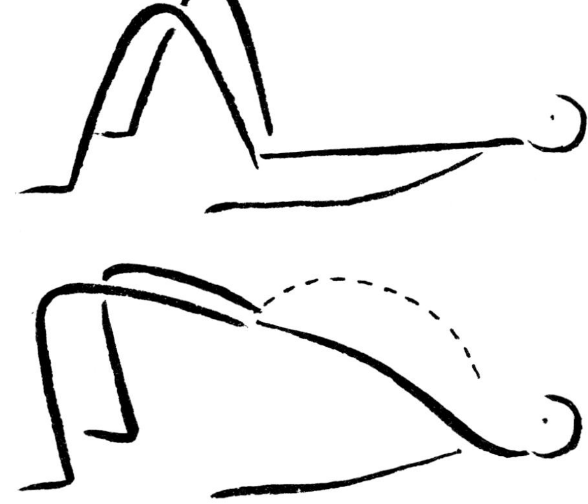

1. Examine drawings of spine on p. 65 and skeleton on p. 48. Lie down on your back. Place feet flat on floor, a foot apart. Relax arms beside the body. Take a few deep breaths.

2. Breathe in, while raising the whole spine off floor one vertebra at a time, until you are resting on the neck vertebrae, back of the head, shoulders and feet. The inhalation should then be complete.

   Breathe out, while lowering spine, vertebra by vertebra, until tailbone returns to floor. The exhalation should be complete.

As you repeat this exercise, you will develop a rhythm of your own, co-ordinating the speed of the spinal movement with the length of your inhalation and exhalation.

1. Breathing

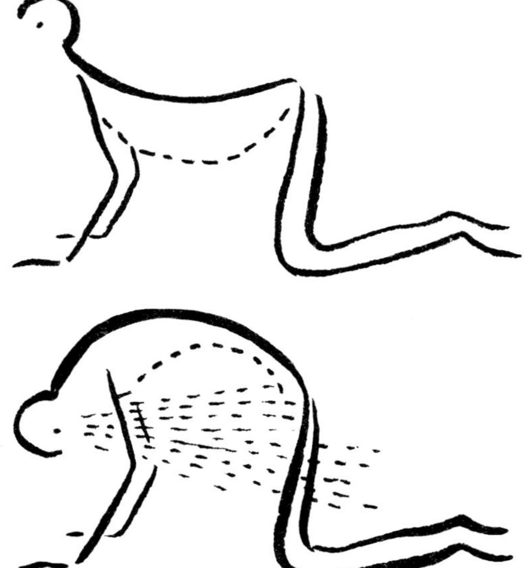

EXERCISE VII

1. Kneel on all fours. Keep arms straight, hands in line with shoulders, knees in line with hips. Hollow the spine, pushing shoulders back, so that stomach drops towards floor. While hollowing spine, breathe in.

2. Pull stomach muscles up, pressing the whole abdomen toward the spine, while breathing out. Make spine as round as possible. Pull chin towards chestbone. Breathe in as above. Return to starting position. Repeat many times.

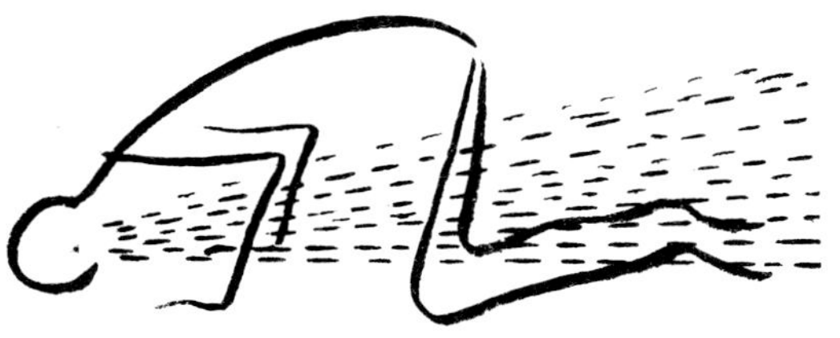

EXERCISE VIII

Kneel on all fours. Place top of head on floor. If possible, do a headstand. If not, look between the knees at wall facing you. Relax stomach muscles and take a deep breath through the nose. Expel air as forcefully as possible through mouth. Direct the outflow of air towards the wall, as if blowing out a candle.

These two exercises especially strengthen muscles that contract the chest and abdomen. It is these muscles that ensure proper exhalation.

EXERCISE IX

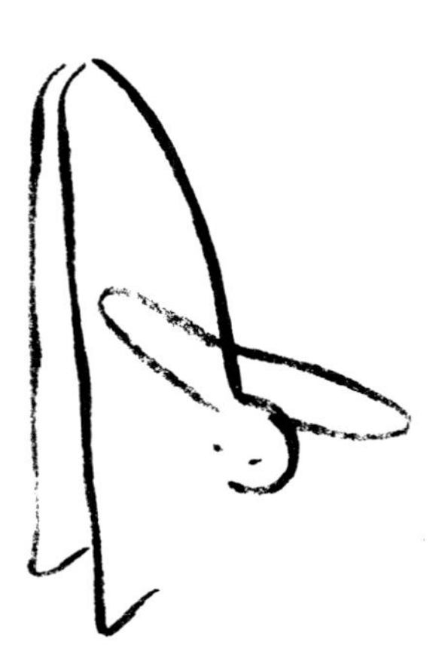

1. Stand with feet a foot apart, toes pointed forward. Hang forward from waist. Interlace fingers behind base of skull.

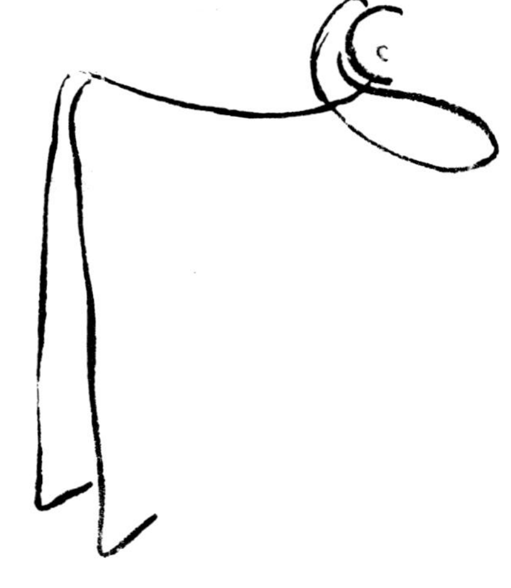

2. Breathe in and lift spine to a horizontal position. Look up. Elbows apart. Breathe out and hang forward. Breathe in and repeat many times.

EXERCISE X

1. Sit on floor, legs straight, feet two or three feet apart. Hands behind buttocks on the floor.

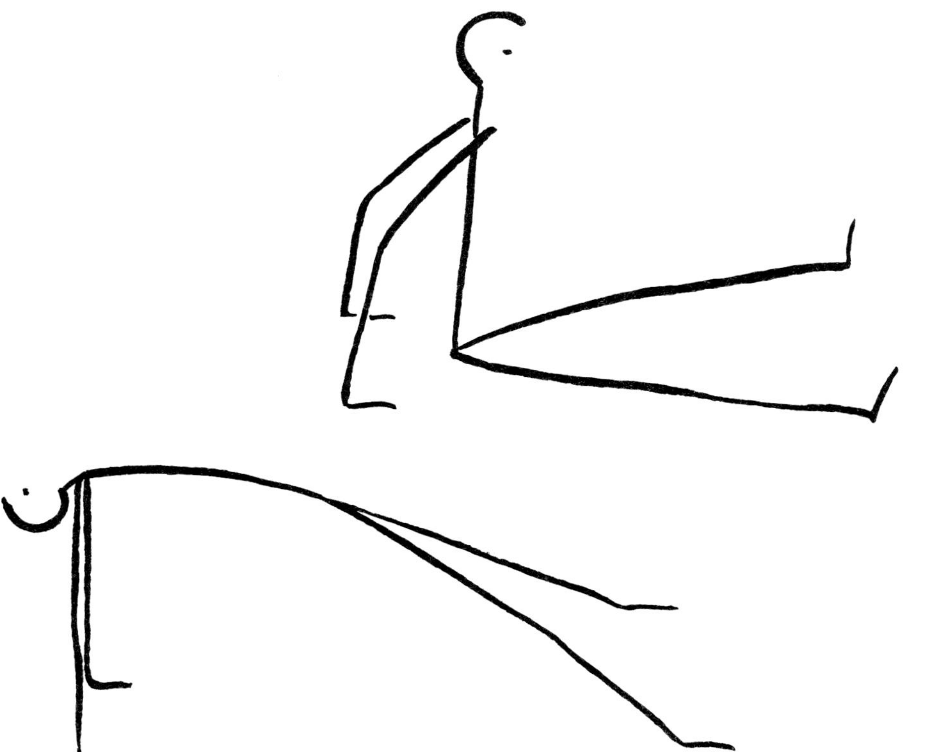

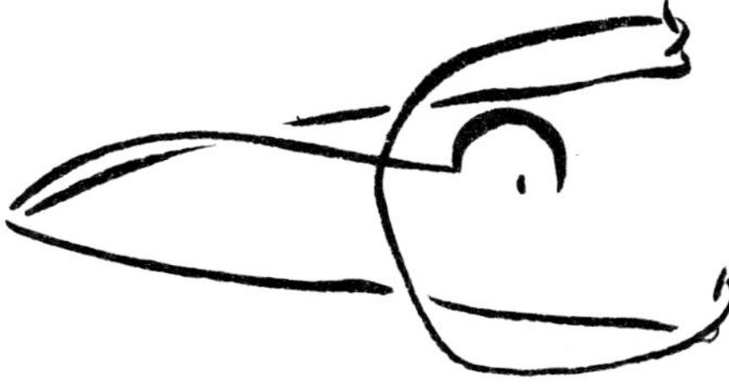

2. Breathing out, lift pelvis off floor, pushing it up as high as possible. Legs straight. Head hanging backwards. Breathing in, return to sitting position.

3. Breathing out, bend forward reaching for toes. Chestbone forward, spine straight, legs straight. Breathing in, return to sitting position.
   Repeat exercise many times.

EXERCISE XI

Lie down on back. Legs straight. Arms over head on floor or next to body or crossed over chest. Breathing out, come up to sitting position and stretch forwards reaching for toes. Remain in forward stretch until exhalation is complete. Breathe in, come up, and lie down. Breathe out and reverse movement. Repeat many times.

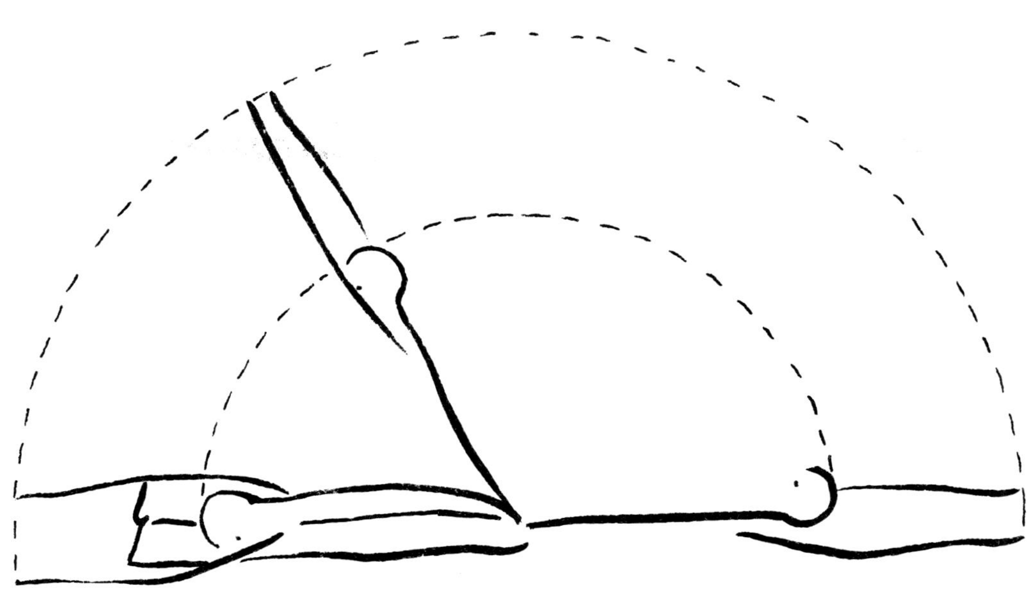

EXERCISE XII: GREETINGS TO THE SUN

Greetings. Light brings life. Life brings growth. Growth brings change. Life is change. An animal's way is known before its birth. A human being can make its own path. Each path is unique – if you feel that way. The path is life. As you explore your body, you will become aware that there is always more energy available – if you will use it. Unused muscle fibres, unused brain cells, unused energy. If you live in a rut, you will slowly lose sight of other ways and other people. Eventually the rut will become so deep, you will need artificial light to illuminate your subterranean passages. Keep the sun in mind. Become aware of your self and your instincts. Do not become trapped in categories, boxes, jobs. Open your self to the world around you. Greetings.

2. Breathe in through nose, stretch up, hang backward.

1. Stand with feet slightly apart, toes pointed forward. Palms together in front of chestbone.

3. Breathe out through mouth, come up, hang forward. Place hands on floor next to outside of feet. Legs straight.

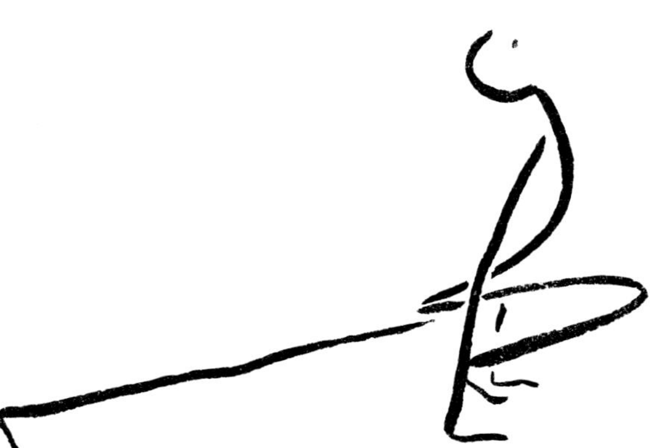

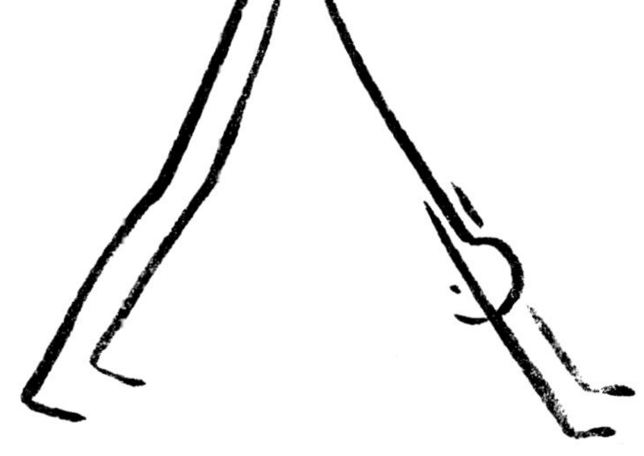

4. Breathe in through nose. Bend left knee and bring left buttock close to left ankle. Stretch right leg back straight. Tuck toes under. Arch spine. Look up.

5. Holding breath, place left foot back next to right foot. Push heels toward floor. Push pelvis backward. Eyes look at navel. This cycle of exercises continues on the next page.

6. Breathe out through mouth. Jump both feet backward. Hands stay in place. The whole body lies flat on floor.

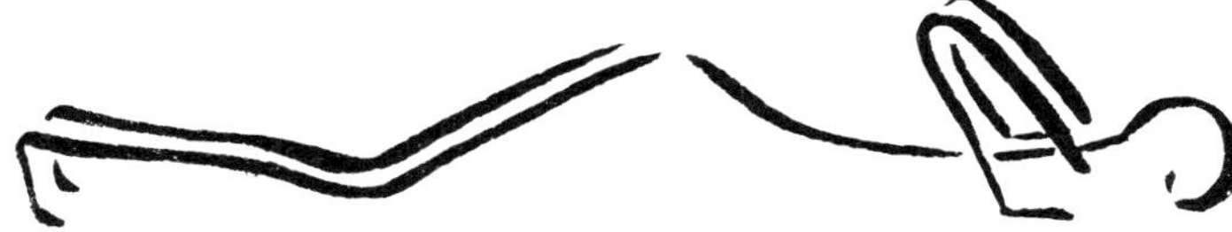

7. Do not yet breathe in. Stay empty. Tuck tailbone upward. Pelvis and thighs come off floor. Forehead on floor. Forehead, hands, chest, knees, and toes contact floor.

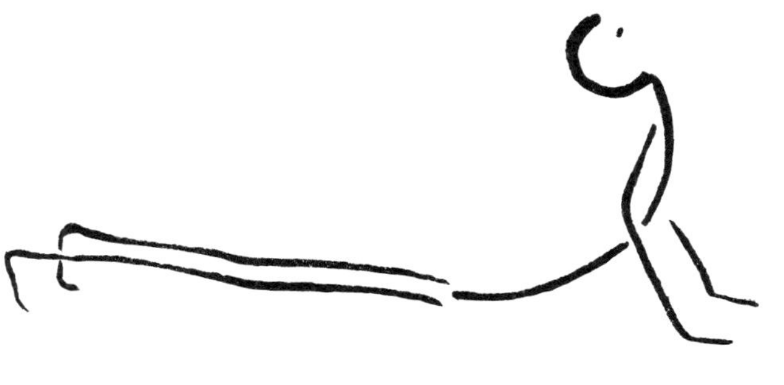

8. Inhale through nose. Place pelvis back on floor again. Push abdomen and chest off floor by straightening arms. Hollow spine, drop head backward. Look up.

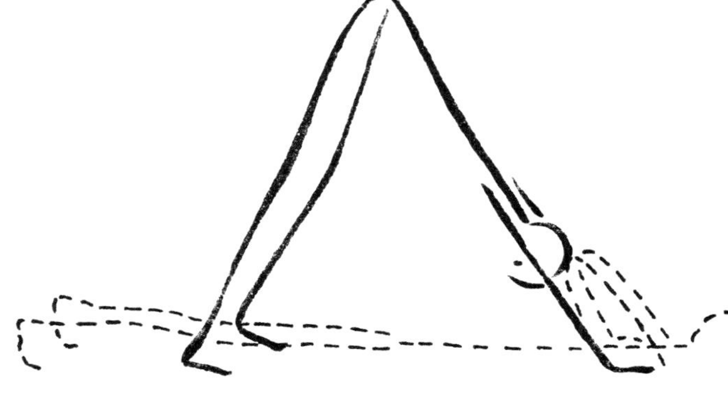

9. Holding breath, go back to standing on hands and toes.

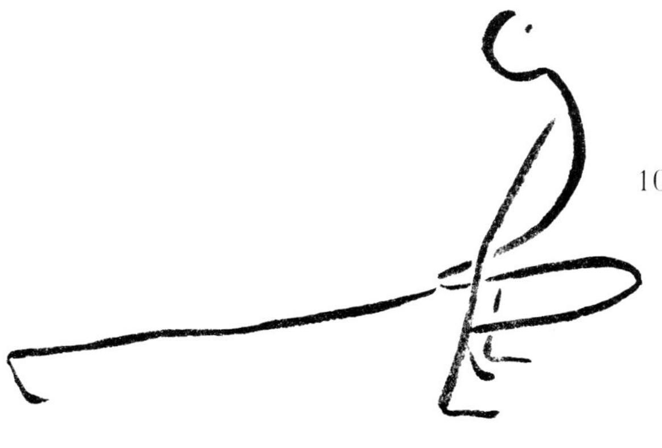

10. Still holding breath, put right foot between hands on floor. Left leg stretches backward. Arch spine. Look up.

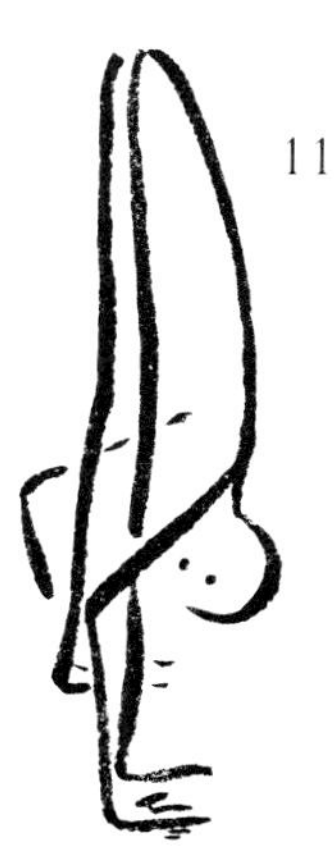

11. Exhale through mouth. Move left foot next to right foot. Straighten legs and hang forward. Inhale through mouth and return to starting position. Repeat whole cycle for three to fifteen minutes.

2. FEET AND HANDS

Both western and eastern medicine recognise that there is a continuous flow of energy within the body: during movement and during rest, from brain to muscles, from nerve to nerve, from organ to organ. The energy flows through the body in definite patterns or zones. When the energy flow is obstructed, we call it disease. Pressure points are places where the energy within the body comes to the surface. They have a particular sensitivity. In case of malfunction, they are quite painful. It follows that treatment for dis-ease is most effective at these points. Practitioners of acupuncture work with some 1000 of these points.

Although pressure points are located all over the body, there is an intense concentration in the feet and hands. Through the ages, study has shown the existence of physical connections between the points in these two areas and the major organs of the body. This science is known as reflexology, as it traces the reflex (movement) involved when pressure points are activated. This chapter deals with these connections in great detail. In the various other chapter introductions, pressure points have been included in drawings of the appropriate areas. These points can always use extra attention and massage.

FOOT MASSAGE

Foot massage requires care and concentration. All present or past dis-ease can be traced in the tenderness of reflex points in the feet. While massaging out all tensions, tender spots, and lumps, you will discover the relationship of the different pressure points to the various parts of the body. Move over the foot with a deep rolling and creeping movement of the thumb, fingers, and knuckles. Dwell on sensitive or painful spots. It is useful to keep handy an object such as a pen with a round tip to reach points where the thumb cannot penetrate deep enough.

Begin with the right foot, representative of the right part of the body. Then move on to the left foot. Compare the different reactions of both feet. You may feel a lot of pain at times; this signifies an area or zone that needs more massage and relaxation. No part of your foot should remain unknown to you, and no spot should remain untreated. When working with the toes, do not be afraid to pull them, rub them, stretch them, and move them firmly in all possible directions – backwards and forwards, clockwise and anti-clockwise. Cracking the toes is also very helpful in freeing the energy flow. Crack the toe joints simply by pressing down on them. Familiarise yourself with the drawings of the feet on the following pages. Although you may begin the massage at any point, we begin with the heel.

Explore your HEELS, the inside and the outside. The reflex points for the *ovaries, testicles, uterus, prostate gland* and reproductive energy in general are situated on the heel and achilles tendon. Deep massage of this area will reveal amazingly sensitive spots. Massage here will have a stimulating and rejuvenating effect on the whole body. These spots may be particularly sensitive for women who are menstruating. Massage will also be especially beneficial in cases of premenstrual tension. Massage in the area for the sexual organs should be followed by a short massage of the kidney reflex point. (See drawing on next page.) On the outside and bottom of the heel are the reflex areas for the *sciatic nerve* and the *hip*.

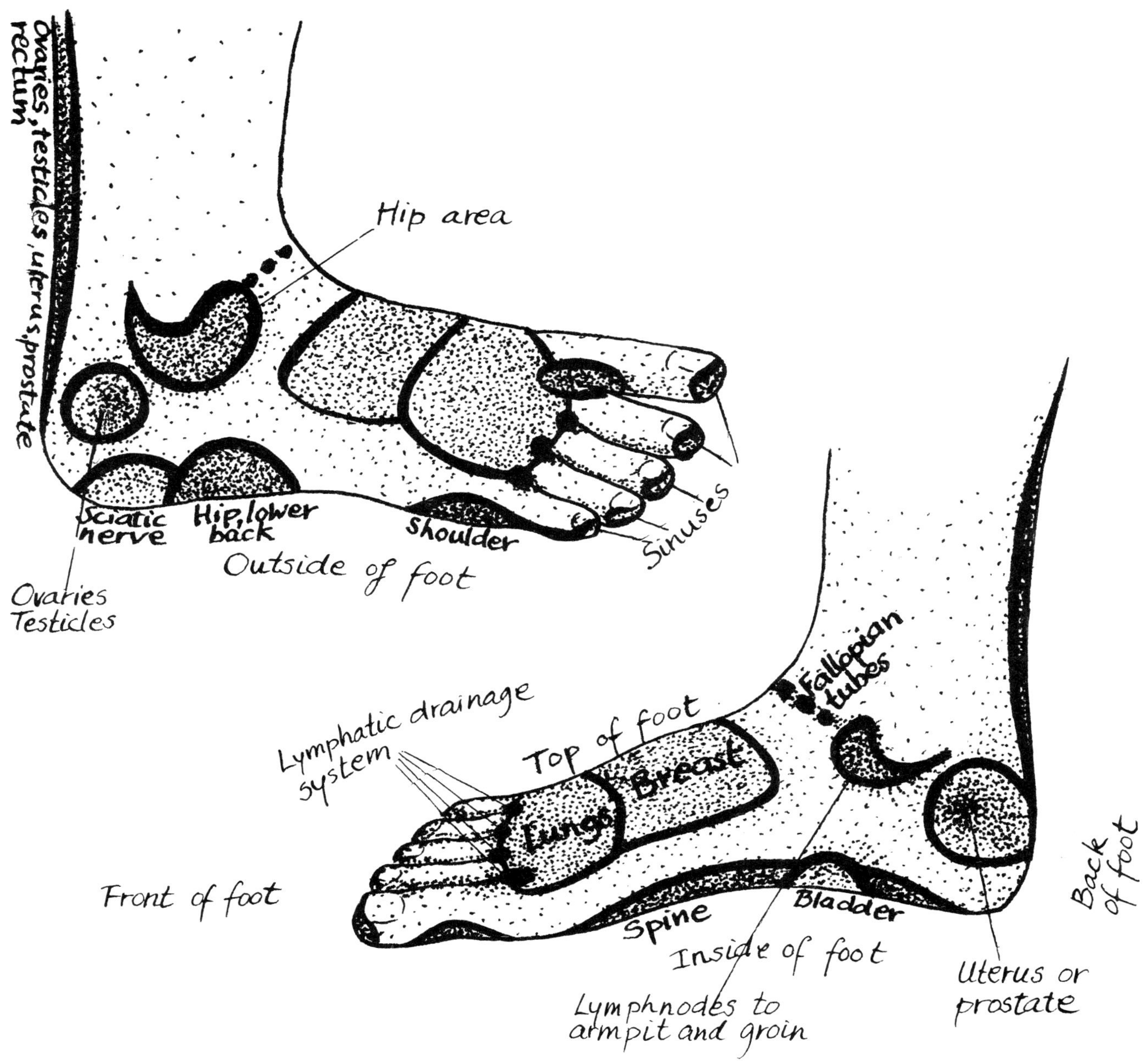

On the TOP of the foot, at the base of each toe you find the pressure points for the *lymphatic drainage system.* The point on the inside of the neck of the big toe usually reveals great sensitivity. Towards the middle are the areas for the *breast* and *lungs*. Over the front of the ankle lie the reflex points for the *fallopian tubes*. On the outside of the ankle, under the ankle bone is the reflex point for the *lymph nodes to armpit and groin.*

The BIG TOE represents the head: the top of the toe, the top of the head; the neck of the toe, the *neck.* Slightly toward the inside on the top of the toe is a very sensitive spot, the reflex points for the *pineal gland.* In the centre of the bottom pad you will find a very small point for the *pituitary gland* – perhaps use a pen tip for this one. The inside of the big toe, next to the second toe, represents the face. Facial tensions will definitely be reflected from this area after deep probing. Massaging the big toe is also extremely beneficial for headaches, tense eyes, and tense ears. The condition of your neck and upper spine will improve if you keep the neck and base of the toe soft and free of tender spots. The *thyroid gland* is represented on the inside of the pad under the

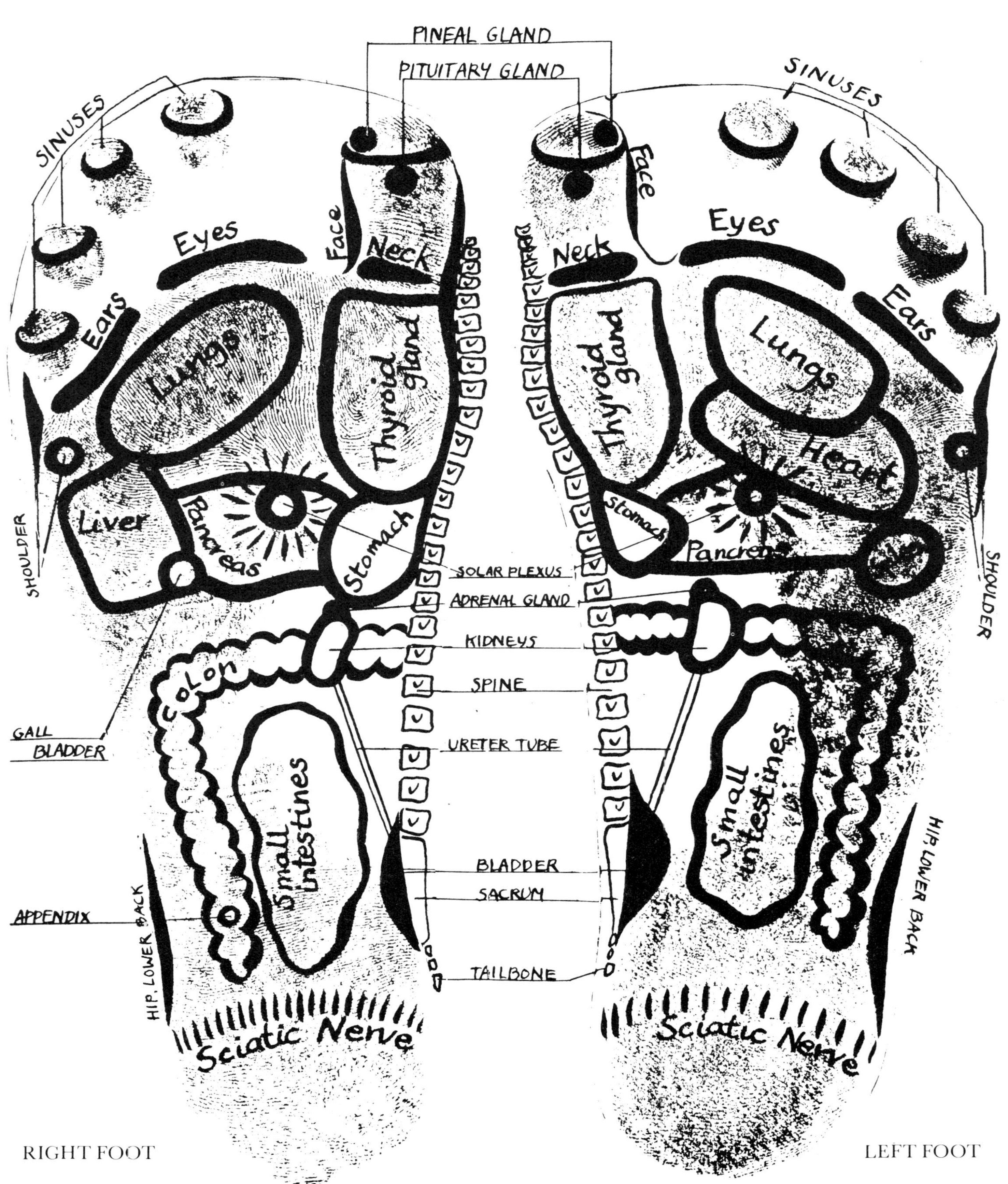

RIGHT FOOT

LEFT FOOT

base of the big toe. Men may need to press more deeply than women in this area. From the neck of the big toe to the inside of the pad under the heel runs the reflex area for the *spine*. Usually pressure on this area feels very pleasant and soothes tired feet. Deep search in this strip will show up weaknesses in your spine.

The SMALL TOES also represent parts of the head. The little pads under the tips of the toes represent the *sinuses*. The reflex points for the *eyes* are found at the base of the second and third toes, for the *ears* at the base of the fourth and fifth toes. Search thoroughly for tender spots here as well as in between the toes. On the outside of the foot just below the little toe is the point for the *shoulder*. As stiff neck and shoulders are often connected with obstructions in the spine, also treat this area.

The BALL of the foot represents the shoulders, upper part of the back, and the chest. In the pad below the second and third toe is situated the *lung* reflex point. Massage quite firmly in this area, trying to reach in between the foot bones. If you have been smoking for many years, you may find small lumps under the skin in this area. In the middle of the lower part of the ball of the foot, you will find the reflex point for the *solar plexus*. Deep pressure here can cause sharp pain. The best way to relax this point is to coordinate massage with breathing. Breathe in deeply while applying pressure, hold for about five seconds, and breathe out while releasing pressure. Repeat several times. Surrounding the solar plexus point is the area for the *pancreas*. Under the base of the little toe in the right foot is the area for the *liver*. You can easily check the condition of your liver by digging your fingers underneath the ribcage on the right side. Sensitivity here will correspond to sensitivity in the foot. Massage the foot with deep rotating movements, touching every possible spot. At the base of the liver area, next to the pancreas area, is the reflex point for the *gall bladder*. In the left foot, corresponding to the liver area on the right foot, is the area for the *spleen*. Check the condition of your spleen by digging your fingers under the left side of the ribs. Also on the left foot, slightly more towards the centre, is the pressure point for the *heart*. Massage here will also affect the arteries and veins round the heart.

The HOLLOW of the foot represents the middle of the body. On the inside of the hollow of the foot, below the big toe, is the reflex point for the *stomach*. Massage with knuckle or thumb from the centre of the foot towards the inside where the spine area is situated, passing under the base of the big toe. Stomach cramps and ulcers will certainly show up here. Throughout the hollow of the foot, you will find reflex points for the *small intestines* and *colon*. Deep pressure, rubbing, and even hitting with the fist will have a very soothing and stimulating effect; your feet will feel warm and glowing. The *kidney* and *adrenal gland* reflex points lie midway down near the inside of the foot. The kidney reflex area is always very sensitive, as it is an organ which eliminates poisons from the system. The *ureter* area is a thin line running from kidney to bladder area. The area for the *bladder* is situated in the inside of the foot next to the pad of the heel. In this area are also located the points for the *tailbone* and *sacrum*. Apply different kinds of pressure, deep and light, moving slowly and carefully over this area.

Each foot massage should end with a massage of the top of the foot. Combining this massage with exercises for the feet and ankles will in a short time produce a new pair of much healthier feet, as well as improving the general health of the entire body.

HAND MASSAGE

The concept and procedure for hand massage are basically the same as for massage of the feet. Examine the diagrams of the hands (overleaf). They show an almost exact correspondence with reflex points of the feet. The thumb, like the big toe, represents the head, including points for the pineal and pituitary glands. Familiarise yourself with these drawings, so that you will be aware of the areas you are affecting during the massage. Fingers and knuckles usually do the work of massage all over the body. Now the 'massagers' also become the 'massaged'. Due to the proliferation of nerve endings in the hands, we have more control over the hands than over the rest of the body put together. Also, the wrists and hands contain 27 different bones. The ability to move and manipulate our fingers and hands is great.

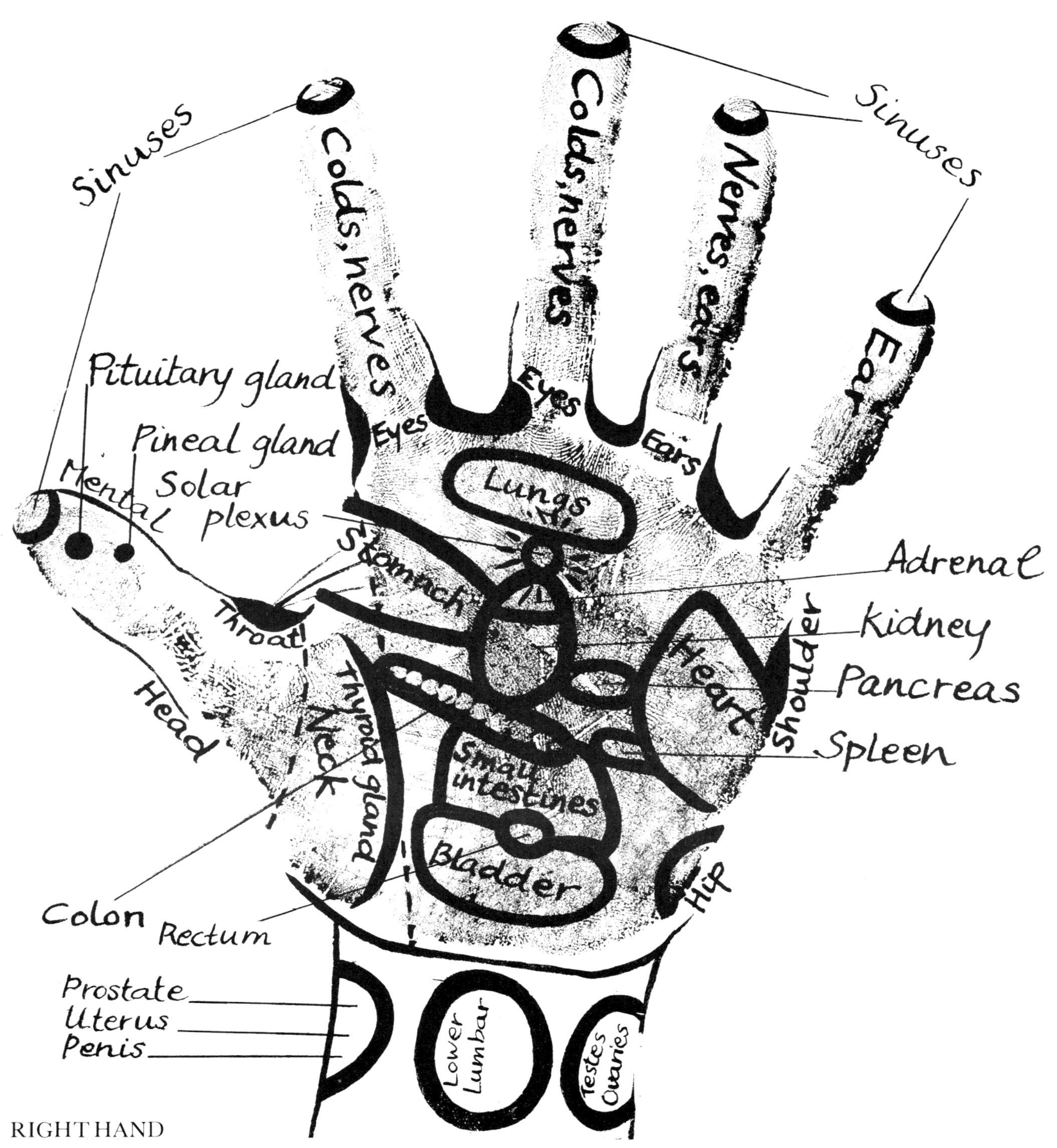

RIGHT HAND

'o begin, shake both hands from the wrist to relax them as much as possible. Starting with the thumb, press the very p between thumb and index finger of the opposite hand. You can draw the nail of the opposite thumb across this tip as ose as possible to, or perhaps slightly under, the nail. Work round the tip of the thumb with a deep rolling movement. 'ontinue downwards on the pad of the thumb, pressing as deeply as possible. Work your way to the base of the thumb, ıen up the sides and down the front. Touch every spot on the thumb: pushing in, stretching, moving clockwise and nti-clockwise. While moving from thumb to index finger, or after working on all of the fingers, pinch and massage the eb between thumb and index finger. You can use either the opposite thumb and finger or the opposite web area – in

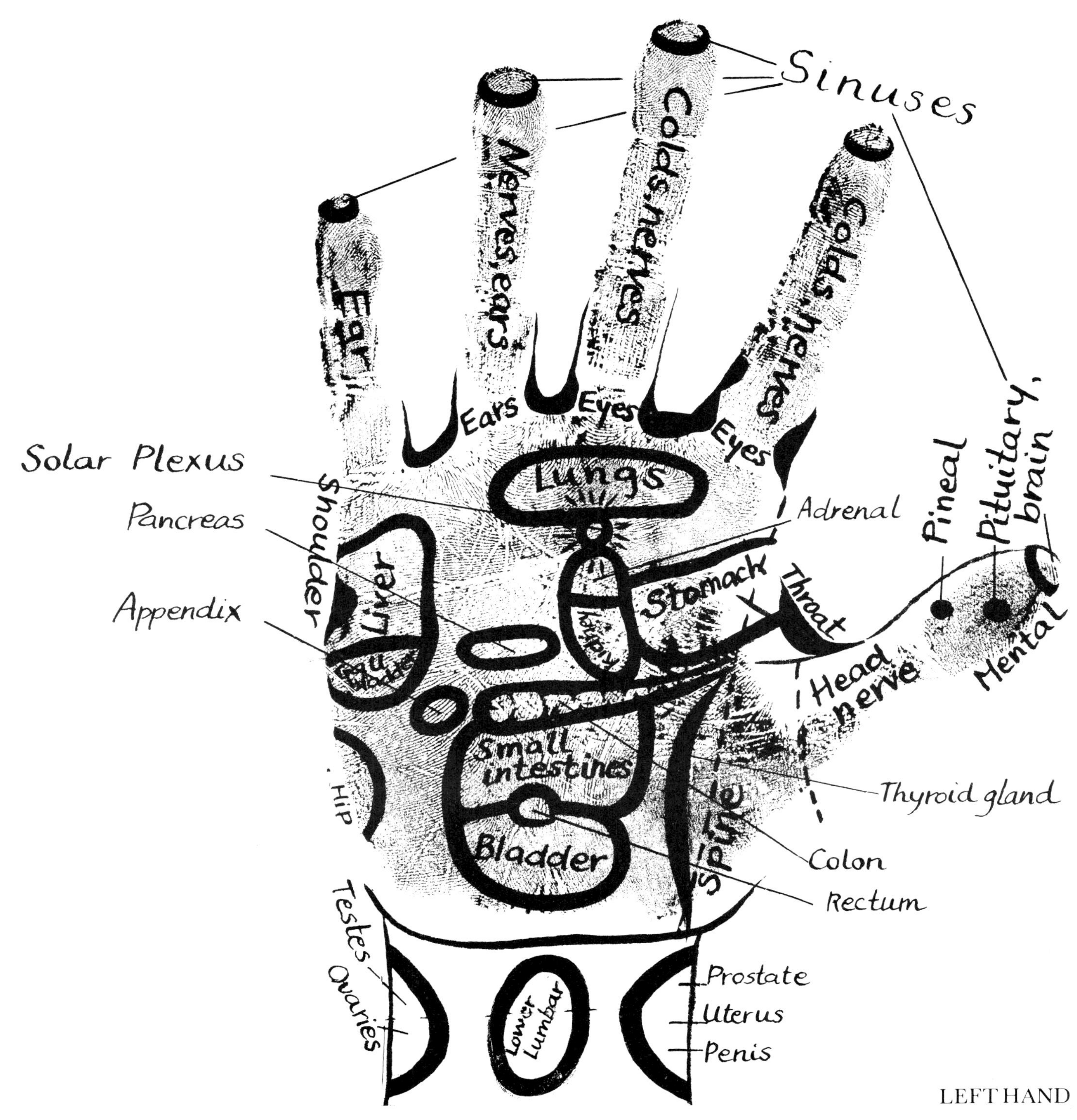

LEFT HAND

which case both webs will be massaged at the same time. Likewise for the webs between the fingers.

One effective technique, especially for the palm area, is to push in simultaneously from both sides of the hand with the thumb and one or two fingers of the opposite. You can thus create an intense concentration of energy between them. As by now you have some experience of working with reflex points, you can create your own movement, focusing on sore spots or small lumps you will encounter, while pressing with enough force to feel the bones and muscles within. As mentioned earlier, you may find the rounded tip of a pen useful as a probe. Remember to massage both hands to maintain the body's balance.

CARE OF THE FEET

The human animal faces the world standing on two feet. In most ordinary positions one or both feet are in contact with the floor, the pavement, or the earth. Feet are something we usually take for granted. They are far removed physically from the eyes and even the hands. The neglect with which we treat our feet is deplorable, especially as the feet mirror all the important organs of the body. Foot aches, blisters, bunions, weak ankles, fallen arches are caused by cramping shoes, high heels, and the like. The tremendous boom in sales of 'support' is due only to the fact that the condition of our feet has deteriorated over the years.

The feet, each of which contains 26 bones (compared with only 4 in the rest of the leg), are not blocks of wood on which we move. They are a sophisticated limb composed of toes, the ball, the hollow, heel, and ankle.

As most of us must wear some kind of shoes in our daily activity, it is important to choose a pair that does not squeeze the big toe against the small toes. The big toe should have the freedom to move away from the little toes. When you stand up, feet together, ankles touching, your two big toes should be in contact up to their tips. Shoes should not restrict independent movement of the little toes. Shoes should allow the weight of the body to rest on the whole of the foot. When you walk, you should be able to feel your weight shifting from the heel, along the outside of the foot, and then diagonally across to the toes, especially the big toes.

Take special care of the soles of the feet. Keep the skin soft. Most chemists sell files to remove callouses and hard patches. After a bath, rub the skin with a slice of lemon or a few drops of cider vinegar. Then massage the skin with a handcream or oil. Good oils are: mustard, which has a penetrating and warming effect; sesame seed oil, which is soothing and has a nutty smell; and wheat germ oil, which is also quite soothing and contains vitamin E. You can scent it yourself with a drop of lemongrass, cinnamon-leaf, or lavender oil.

EXERCISE I

1. Sit on floor, putting hands behind you, palms down on the floor. Relax legs, keeping them parallel. Bend knees. Cross left leg over right leg. (Second picture below and first picture on next page show right leg over left.)

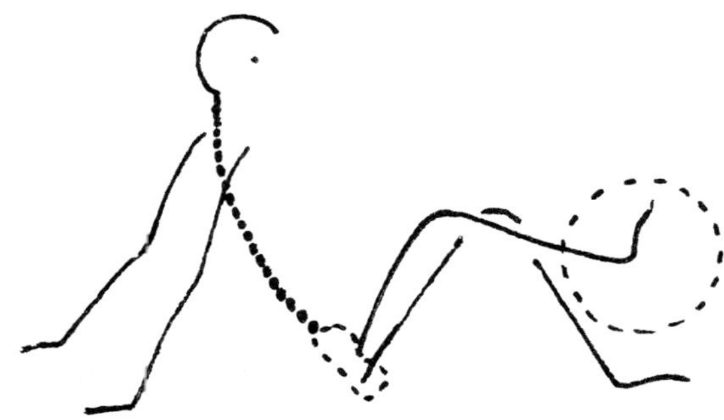

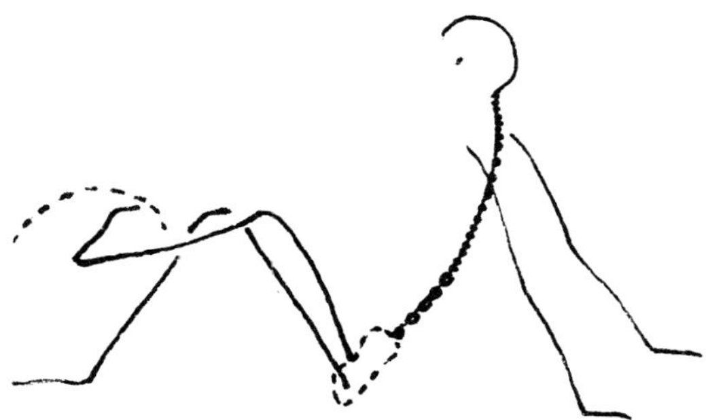

2. Turn ankle in a slow circular movement, clockwise and anti-clockwise. If necessary, use your hand to get movement started.

3. Pull foot up, so as to push heel away from, and toes towards, the knee. Then push foot down so that toes point away from body. Repeat many times.

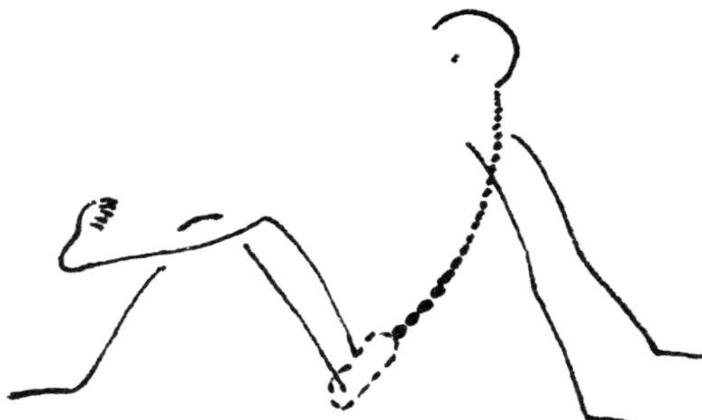

4. Now pull only the toes up towards the body. Hold.

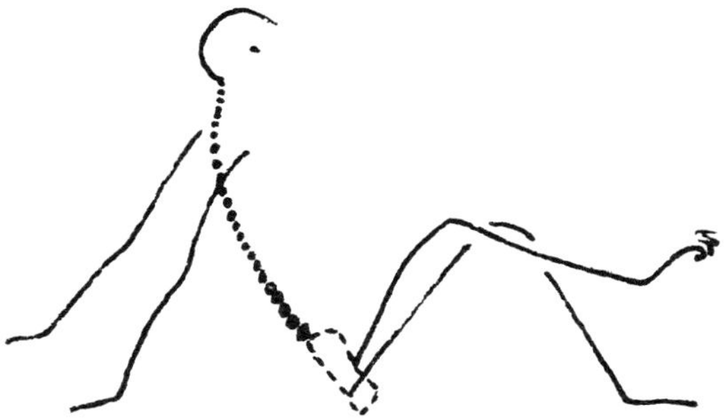

5. Curl toes and make a tight fist with the foot. Hold. Repeat steps 4 and 5 many times. Then repeat steps 2 to 5 with other foot.

EXERCISE II

1. Sit on floor. Place soles of the feet together.

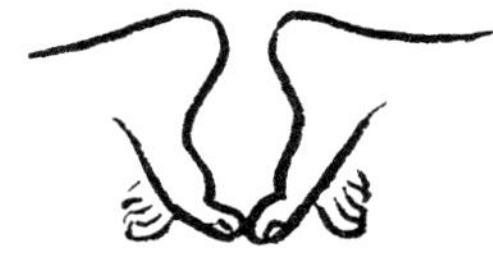

2. Move big toes towards each other and small toes away from each other.

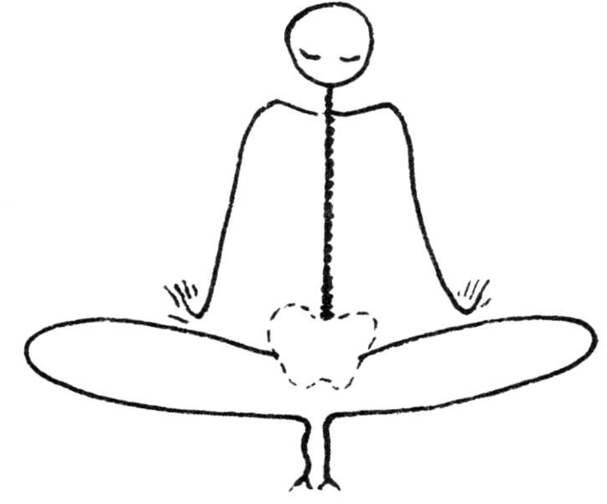

3. Then move big toes away from each other and small toes together.

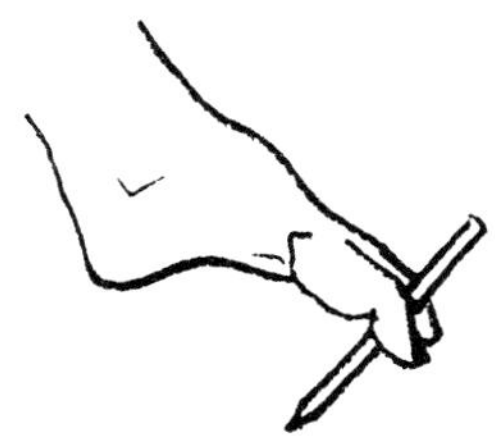

4. Pick up a pencil with the toes. Draw and write with it. Repeat with other foot.

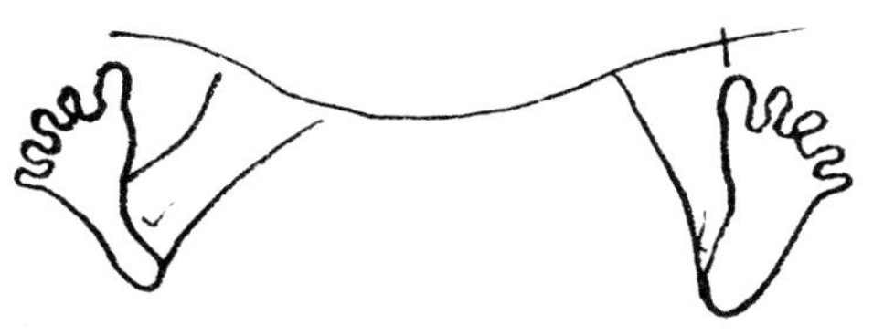

5. Spread all the toes apart. Relax. Repeat many times.

EXERCISE III

1. Sit on floor. Bend left leg and put left arm inside left thigh and under left calf, so that left hand holds lower leg above ankle. Right hand holds inside of lower leg. While shaking foot vigorously, foot and ankle must be completely relaxed.

2. Then rest left leg (above ankle) on right thigh. With left hand hold ankle in place on thigh. With right hand turn left foot in as wide a circle as possible, clockwise and anti-clockwise.

3. Still holding ankle down, use right hand to pull foot towards you and push it away, keeping it parallel to floor. Repeat until ankle feels loose.

4. Place right hand under (top of) left foot. With left hand press down on inside ball of foot. With right hand lift outside of foot so that foot twists and the sole faces the ceiling. Then reverse hands, twisting foot so sole faces the floor.

5. Raise left leg, so that lower part of leg is parallel to floor. Rest heel in left hand and move foot from right to left and back to the right with right hand. Repeat exercise with other foot.

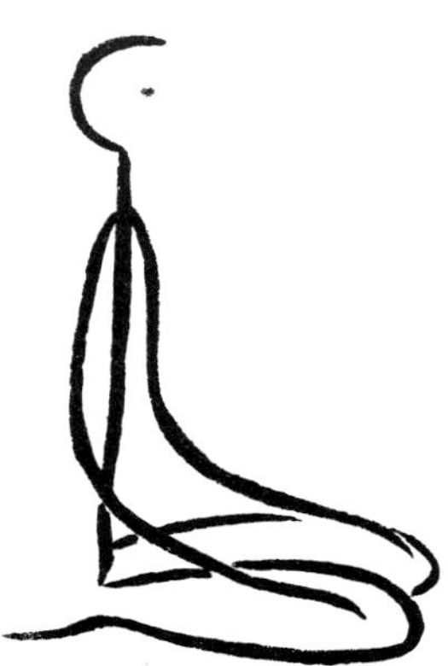

6. Sit on heels. Heels are under buttocks. Hold as long as comfortable.

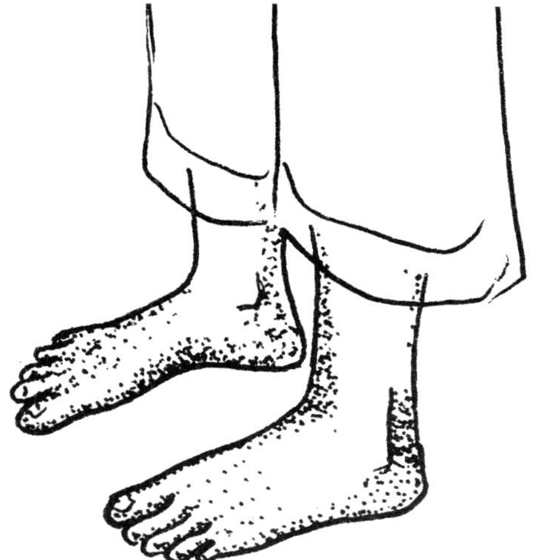

The black areas indicate the foot, or part of foot, to be slapped against the floor.

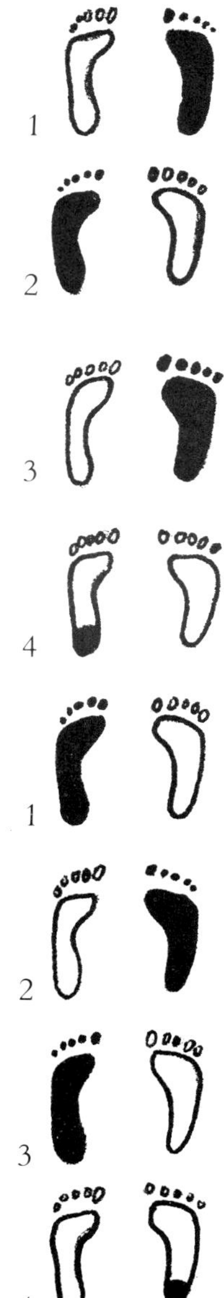

EXERCISE IV: INDIAN DANCE STEP

1. Stand on a smooth floor. Keep feet a fist's width apart, toes pointed forward. Lift right foot off floor. Slap foot back down with force. If foot is relaxed, it will make a clapping sound against the floor.
2. Lift left foot in same way and slap it down.
3. Lift right foot and slap it down.
4. Lift left foot again, but only hit floor gently with heel.
1. Immediately following step 4 above, start sequence again by slapping down the whole of the left foot,
2. then the right foot,
3. then the left foot,
4. then only the right heel.

The hardest slap comes on the count of one. The whole body remains still and relaxed. Eyes remain fixed on a reference point at eye height. Slap feet down as hard as possible, but keep pace steady. Feel whether there is any difference between right and left foot. Make movement from ankles. Continue as long as possible. Remain on the same spot. After some practice you can reach a speed of four slaps per second for about fifteen minutes. This exercise is excellent for coordination and relaxation of the feet, loosening the ankles, strengthening thigh muscles, and improving posture.

3. HAMSTRING AND LEG MUSCLES

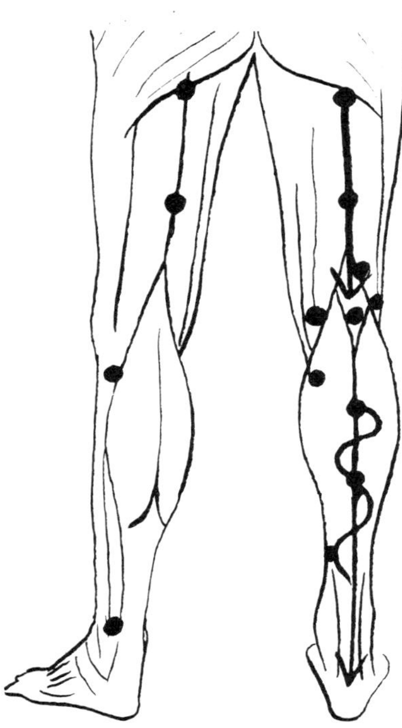

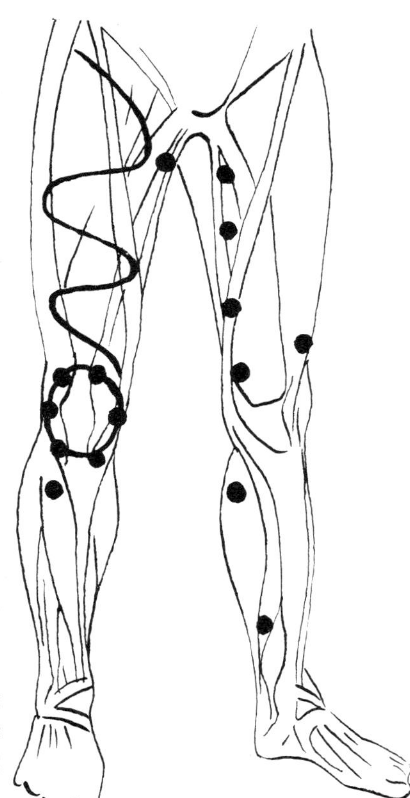

Erect man's original and natural form of movement was, and still is, the legs. But as our society 'progresses', ever more sophisticated means of avoiding using our legs have been developed. Because we often need to travel great distances for work, pleasure, or shopping, we seem not to have the time to walk. For many people, walking or running a mile or two at a stretch produces a great strain on the muscles and tendons. To understand what produces this strain, consider that a muscle is composed of thousands of muscle fibres. Repeated running, especially if muscles are unaccustomed to the task, causes fibres that usually contract to overwork, as well as activating other fibres that are ordinarily latent. What you feel as fatigue is a concentration of sarcolactic acid, a byproduct of muscle activity. As the muscles strain, this acid, which is usually swept away in the blood or oxidised back into the cells to begin the contractile cycle again, accumulates. As breathing has also been strained, the flow of blood through the capillaries adjoining the muscle fibres is disturbed. To reduce this fatigue, massage the area firmly. Gently contract and release the muscle to quicken circulation and thus remove the acid via lungs, kidneys, and other organs. Even professional athletes use only 30 to 35 per cent of the energy liberated in muscle fibres for work. So, we all have a long way to go in learning to make use of our body's energy resources.

You may find the stretching muscles quite painful, especially in the hamstrings (back of the legs), as these muscles are used so infrequently. Remember to work at your own pace. It is only the individual who will know what is most beneficial or most satisfying. The following is a technique for massage of strained muscles.

EXERCISE I

1. Lie down, both legs against a wall. Buttocks and legs in contact with wall. In steps 2 and 3, remember to keep legs straight.

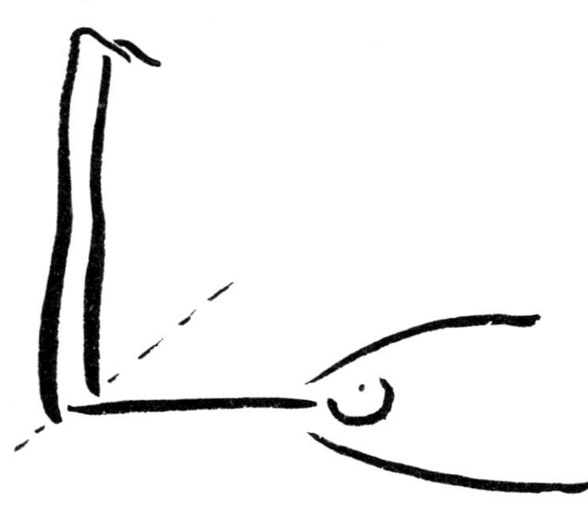

2. Pull right leg towards face with right hand: back and rest of body relaxed. Maintain stretch. Massage back of leg with oil. Rub over muscles; hit gently with fist; knead, and stroke. Hold three minutes. Do not strain. Repeat with left leg.

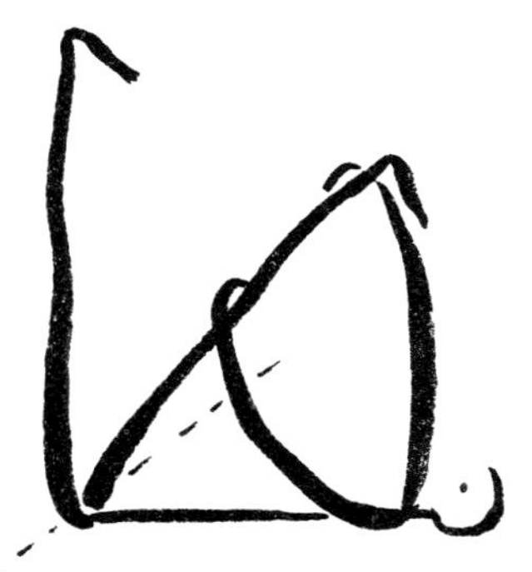

3. Begin as in picture 1. Spread legs, dropping them outward. Relax and feel the pull of gravity. Massage insides of thighs and knees. Hold three minutes.

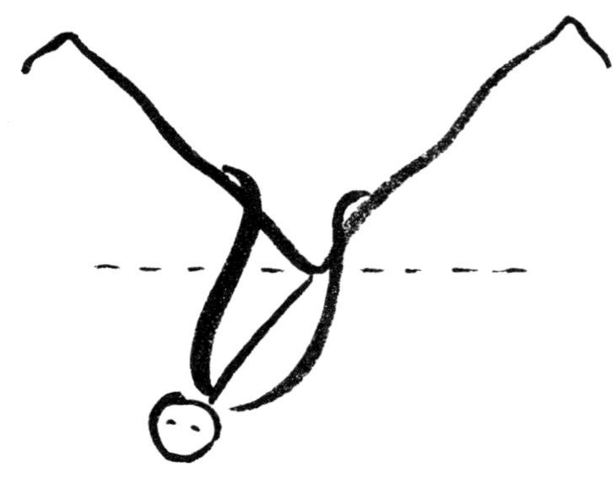

EXERCISE II

Lie down on floor, legs relaxed. Hook index and middle fingers of right hand round right big toe. Raise and then straighten right leg. Stretch heel towards ceiling. Left leg and rest of body relaxed. Turn leg in circles, clockwise and anti-clockwise. Repeat with other leg.

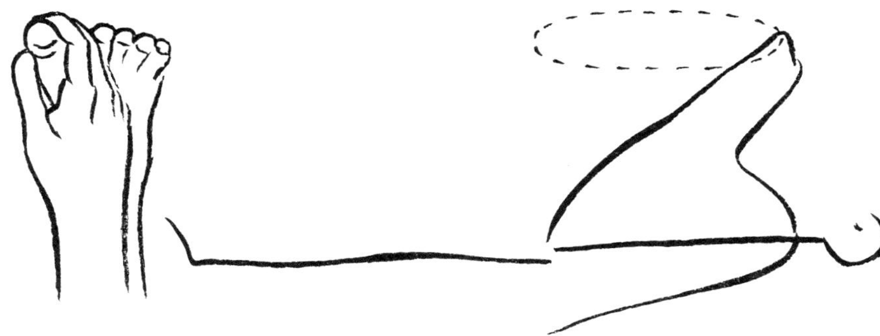

EXERCISE III

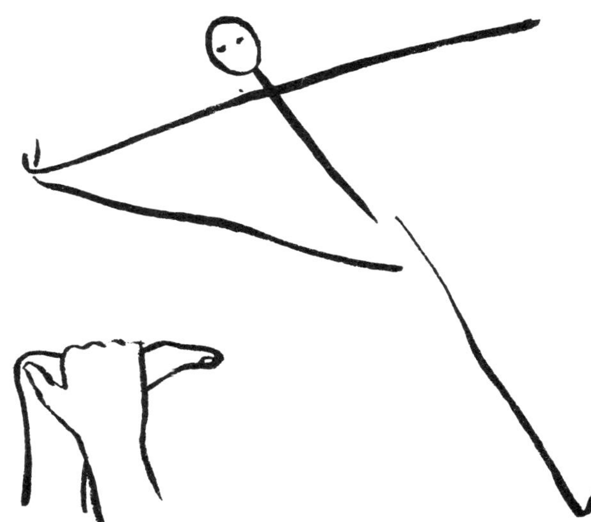

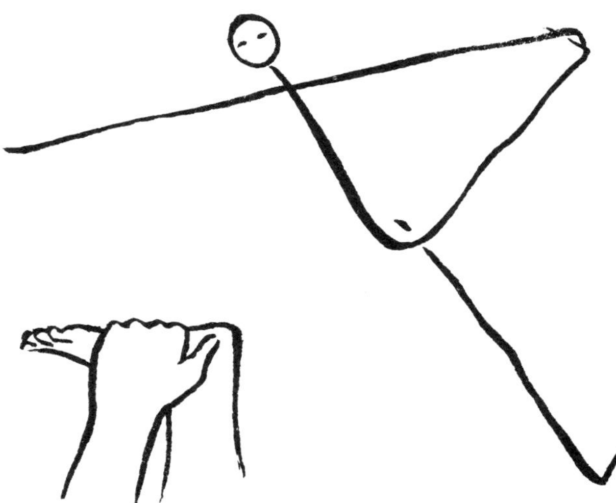

1. Lie down. Right hand holds inside of right foot. Left leg relaxed. Left arm sideways in line with shoulders. Straighten right leg; stretch heel up, away from body. Then drop leg sideways to right, keeping it suspended above floor. Keep left buttock and shoulder in contact with floor.

2. Keeping leg straight, bring it back up. Then hold outside of right foot with left hand. Move right foot to floor on left side of body. Keep right shoulder on floor. Bring leg back up. Shifting hands, move leg to right and left many times. Repeat with other leg.

EXERCISE IV

1. Lie on left side, so that body, legs, and elbow form a straight line. Support head with left hand. Bend right leg and hook two fingers of right hand round big toe. Body and leg should now be in position as in dotted line.

2. Stretch right leg upward. Keep left leg in line with back. Push the right hip forward. Hold. Release and repeat with other leg.

3. Hamstring and Leg Muscles

EXERCISE V

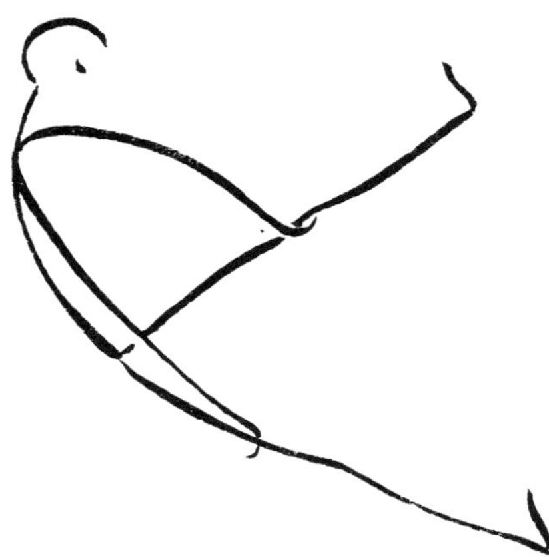

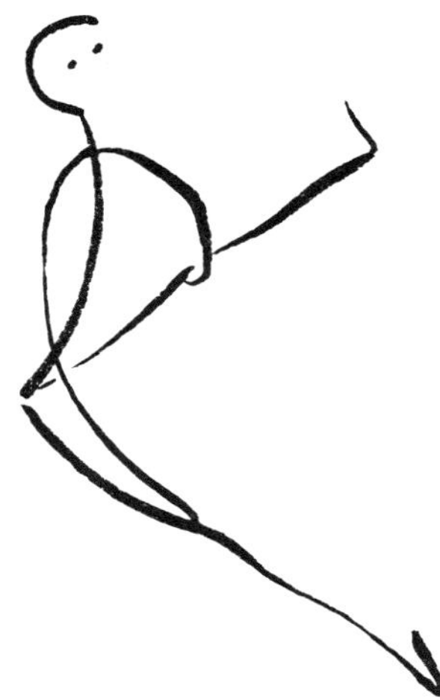

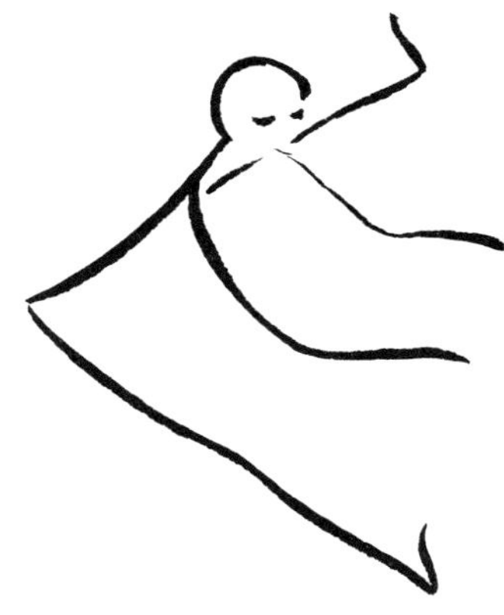

1. Familiarise yourself with skeletal drawings on p. 48. Then sit on floor, spreading legs as far apart as possible. Legs straight. Hands hold insides of knees. Rock pelvis backward, sit on tailbone. Round the spine.

2. Then rock pelvis forward. Sit on sitting bones. Hollow the spine. Repeat many times.

3. Sit on sitting bones. Bend forward from the hips. Place hands as far forward as possible on floor in front of you. Keep spine straight. Move trunk forward and touch floor with elbows. Hands keep moving forward. Repeat many times.

EXERCISE VI

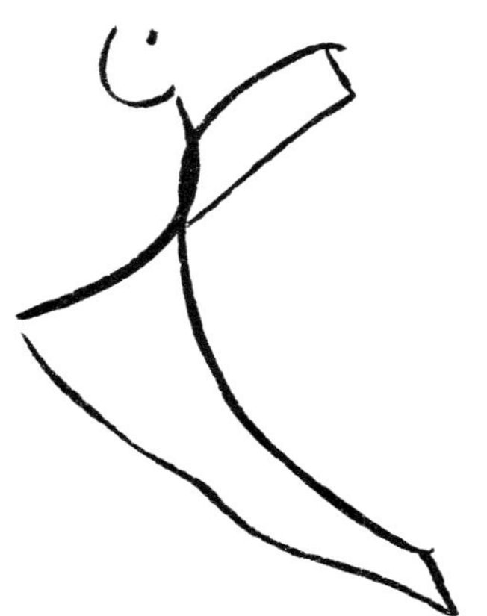

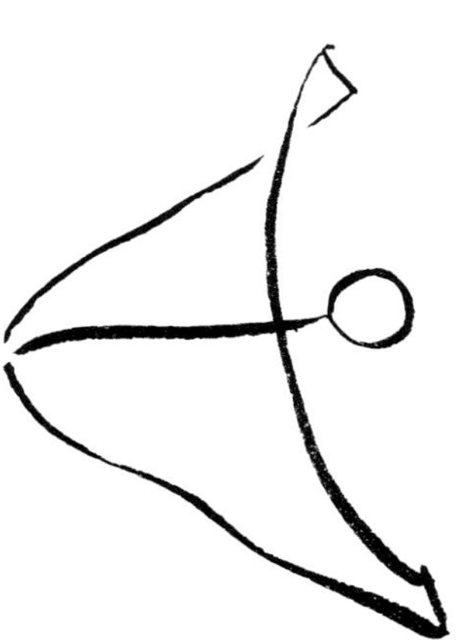

1. Hold both big toes as shown at top of p. 29. Arch the spine. Look up.

2. Stretch chin and chestbone forward and bend forward. Chestbone will eventually touch the floor.

3. Hamstring and Leg Muscles

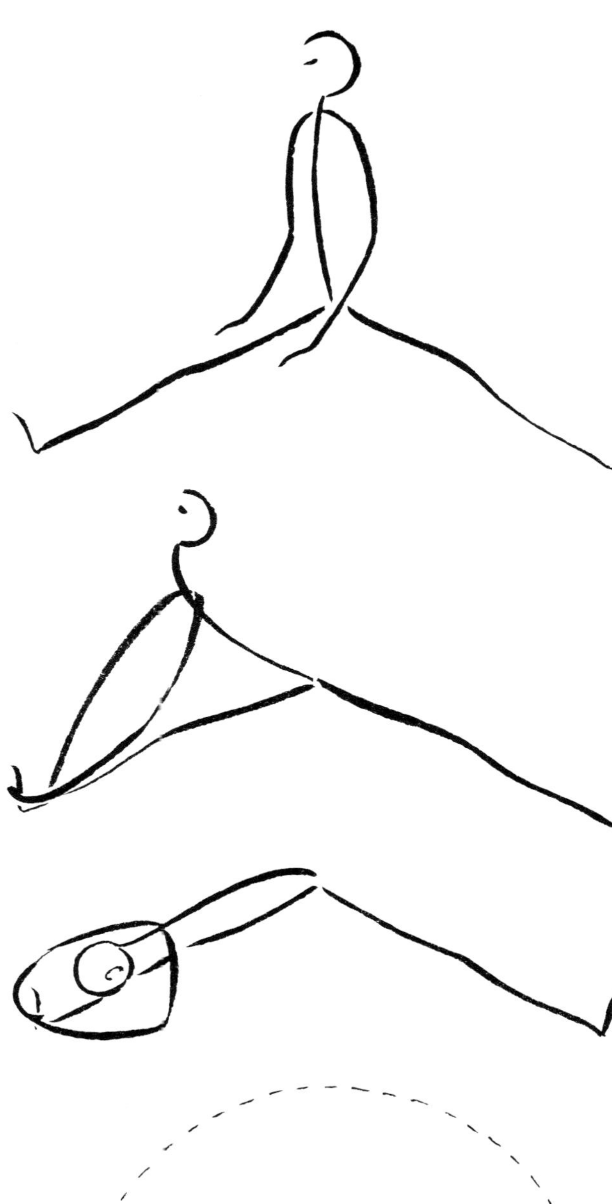

EXERCISE VII

1. Sit on floor. Legs straight and as wide apart as possible. Sit on sitting bones. Twist trunk, and face right foot. Keep spine straight.

2. Left hand reaches forward and holds on to back of knee, calf, ankle, or right foot. Right hand follows but left hand stretches furthest. Hollow spine. Look up.

3. Pull chestbone towards knee. Keep spine straight. Relax and hold. Repeat steps 1-3 on other side.

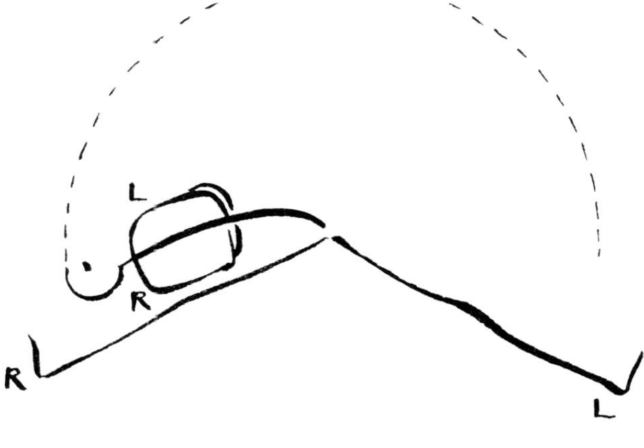

4. Begin again. Keeping legs apart, bring arms behind back and hold on to elbows. Bounce right shoulder toward right knee, while twisting spine so that left shoulder moves backward. Look up at ceiling. Then repeat movement on left side. Then swing from right to left and back, until movement is flowing.

5. Place right elbow on inside of right knee, top of hand on floor. Now tuck hand under calf, ankle; or, if possible, hold foot with thumb over arch, four fingers on hollow of foot. Left shoulder moves backward. Stretch left arm over ear towards right foot. Look up in front of left arm. Right shoulder moves inside right leg. Left buttock on floor. Relax and hold. Repeat on other side.

3. Hamstring and Leg Muscles

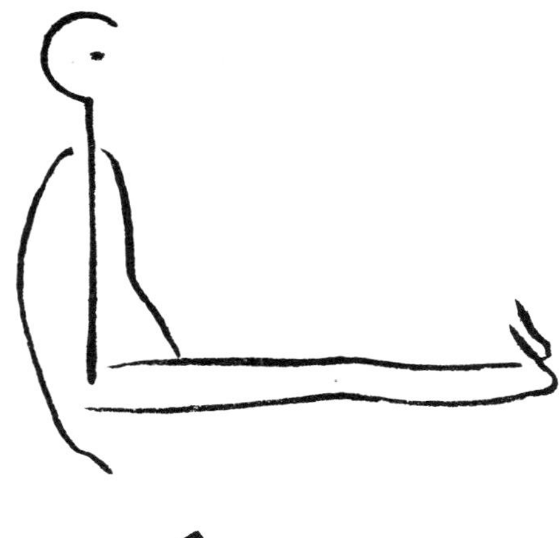

EXERCISE VIII

1. Sit on floor. Legs together and straight, big toes touching. Move toes towards face, heels away from body. With both hands pull the buttock muscles and thigh muscles outward. This will relax buttocks, thighs, and anus. Then tilt pelvis forward, moving tailbone backward. Sit on sitting bones, not on tailbone. Keep spine straight. Move base of skull toward ceiling.

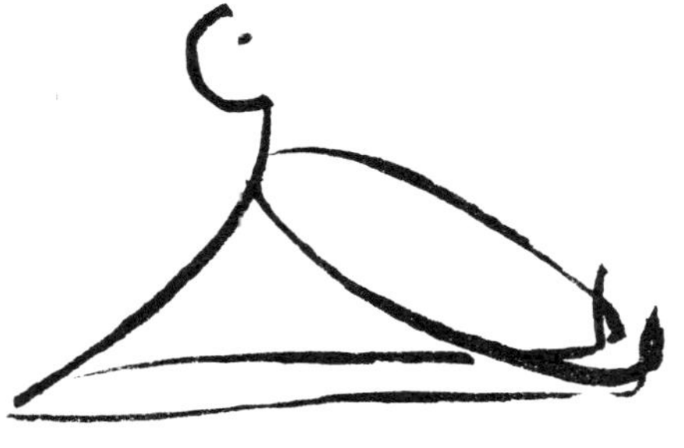

2. Keep spine straight while bending forward. Hold on to back of knees, calves, ankles, or feet with hands. Then hollow spine, looking upward.

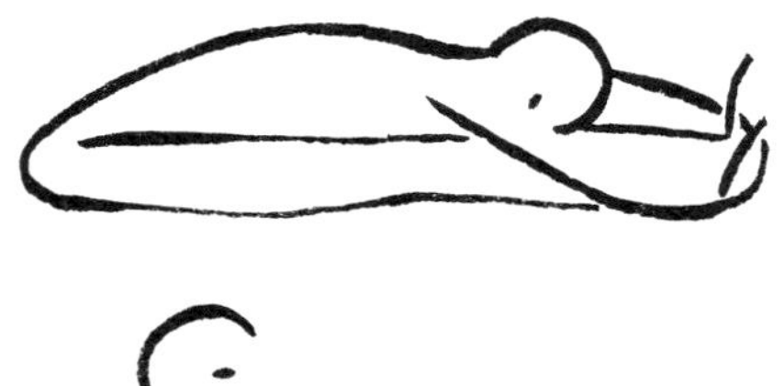

3. Then pull chestbone forward until stomach, chestbone, and head lie on legs. The whole body is relaxed. During this movement, thigh joints turn outward to move knees slightly inward. Tailbone tucks backward. Chin stretches forward, not downward.

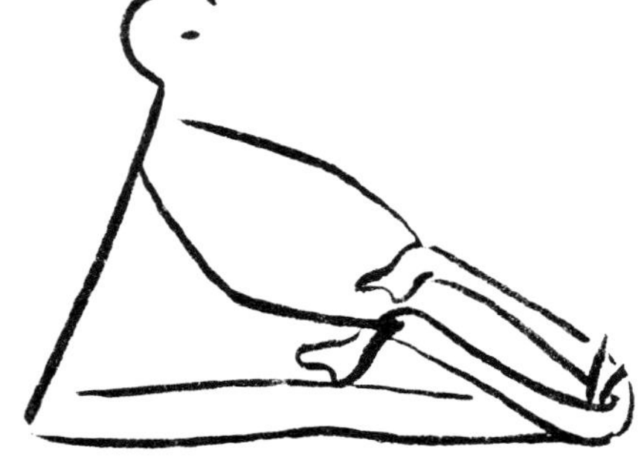

4. If your hamstring muscles are short and tight, it may at first be impossible to sit on sitting bones. If so, loop a scarf or belt around soles of feet. Gently pull forward, keeping spine straight.

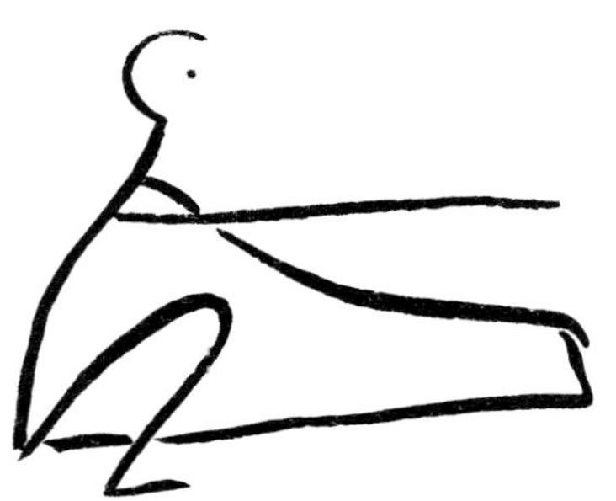

EXERCISE IX

Place right foot flat on floor as close as possible to right buttock. Toes pointed forward. Left hand holds on to left ankle or foot. Keep left leg straight. Stretch right arm forward. Shift weight of body forward and lift buttocks and left leg off floor. Sit back down again. Repeat many times.
Repeat with left foot.

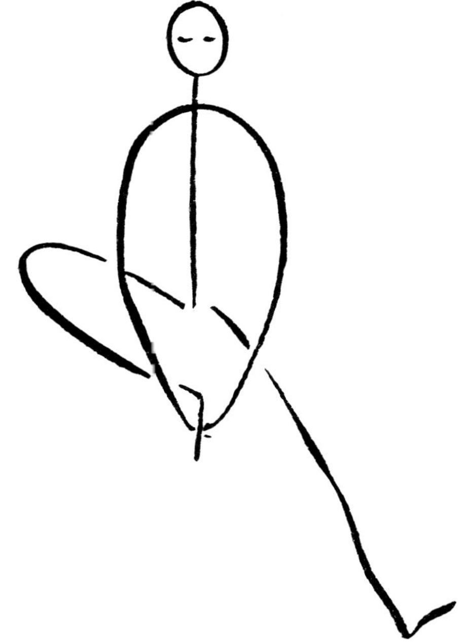

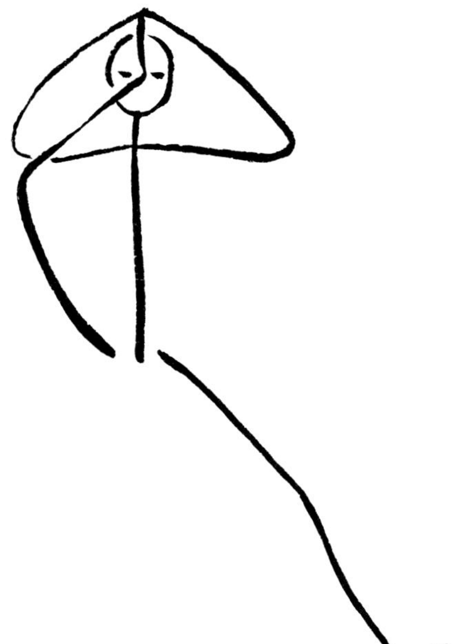

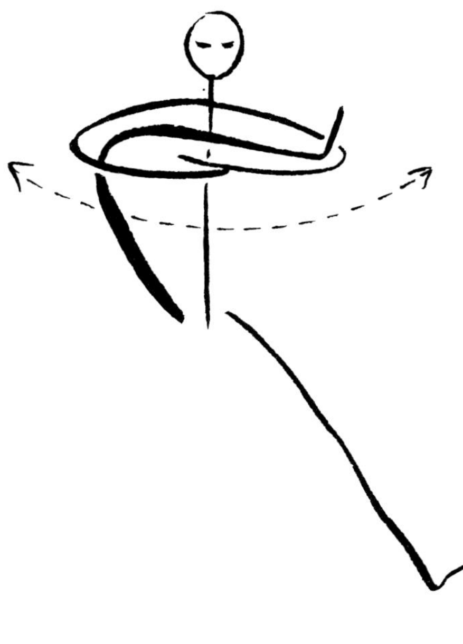

EXERCISE X

1. Sit on floor. Both hands hold right foot. Keep left leg straight Keep spine straight.
2. Then pull foot toward forehead; further to top of the head; further behind head. Then repeat with left foot.
3. Then rest sole of right foot inside left elbow. Rest right knee inside right elbow. By raising left elbow, pull right foot toward left shoulder. Rock leg from right to left and back many times. Repeat with other leg.

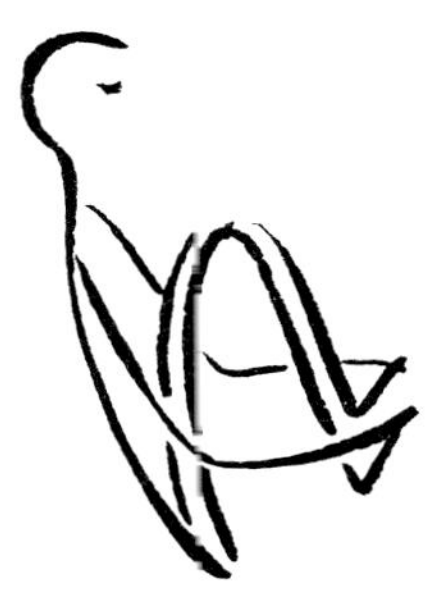

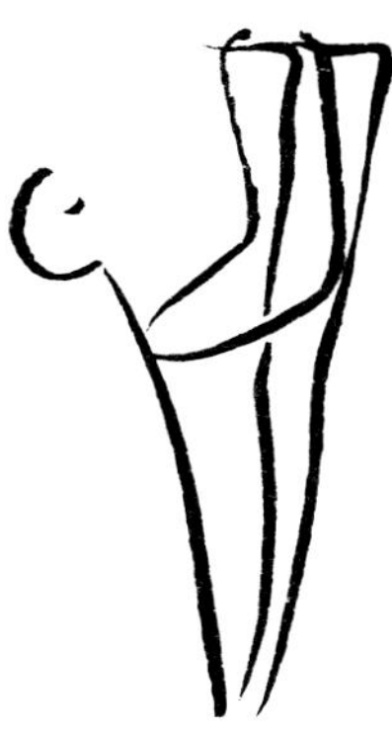

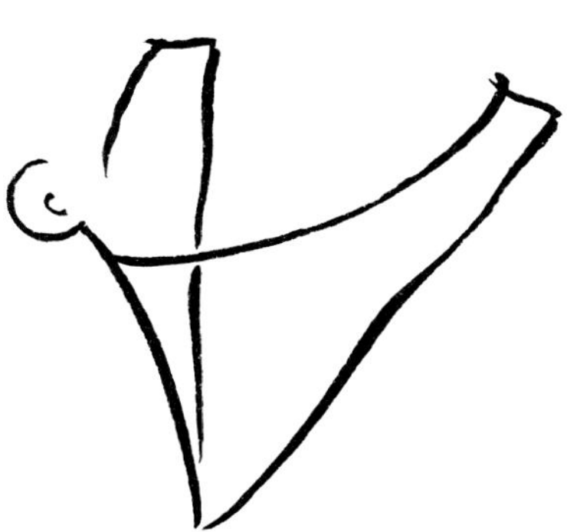

EXERCISE XI

1. Sit on floor. Pull knees toward chest. Hands hold feet
2. Stretch both legs up and balance on sitting bones and tailbone. Keep spine straight.
3. While balancing on tailbone, spread legs and drop them outward. Hold.

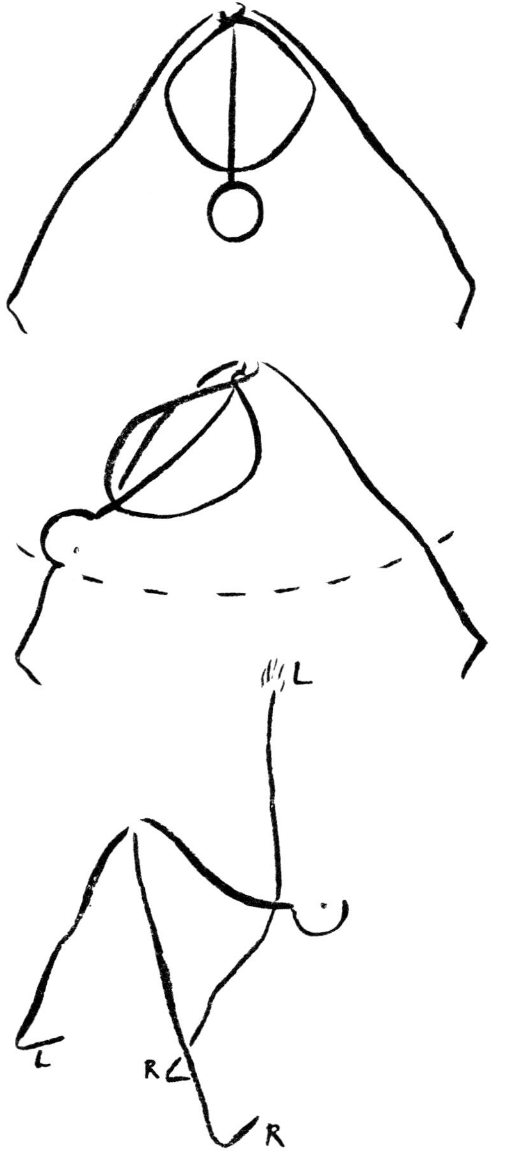

EXERCISE XII

1. Stand with feet two to three feet apart, toes pointed forward. Hands behind lower back. Hold on to one wrist. Hang forward from hips, keeping back straight. Tilt pelvis forward, so tailbone and buttocks move upward. Bounce gently from hips. Repeat many times. Then hang forward again.

2. Using tailbone as a pivot point, move the trunk (bouncing slightly) from left to right and back again, describing as wide an arc as possible.

3. Stand as above. Place right palm between feet on floor, or stretch right hand toward floor. Fingers pointed forward. Twist trunk, moving left shoulder backward. Stretch left arm upward and look straight past thumb of left hand. Palm of this hand should face to the left.
   Repeat with other hand.

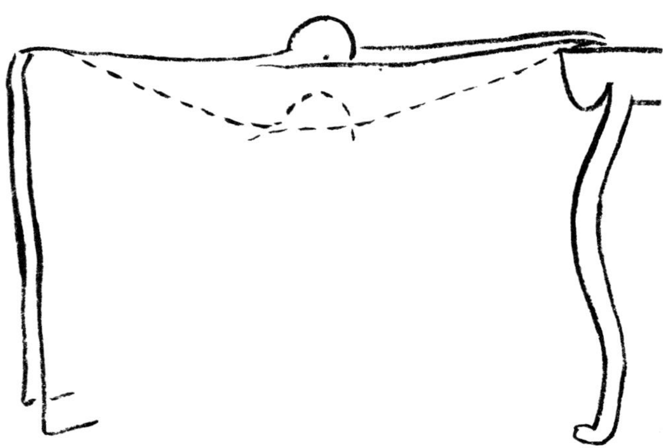

EXERCISE XIII

1. Stand two to three feet away from a table. Place both hands in line with shoulders on edge of table. Back and arms horizontal and straight. Legs straight.

2. Gently bounce chest and armpits towards floor. Move buttocks and tailbone upward. Relax stomach and diaphragm muscles.

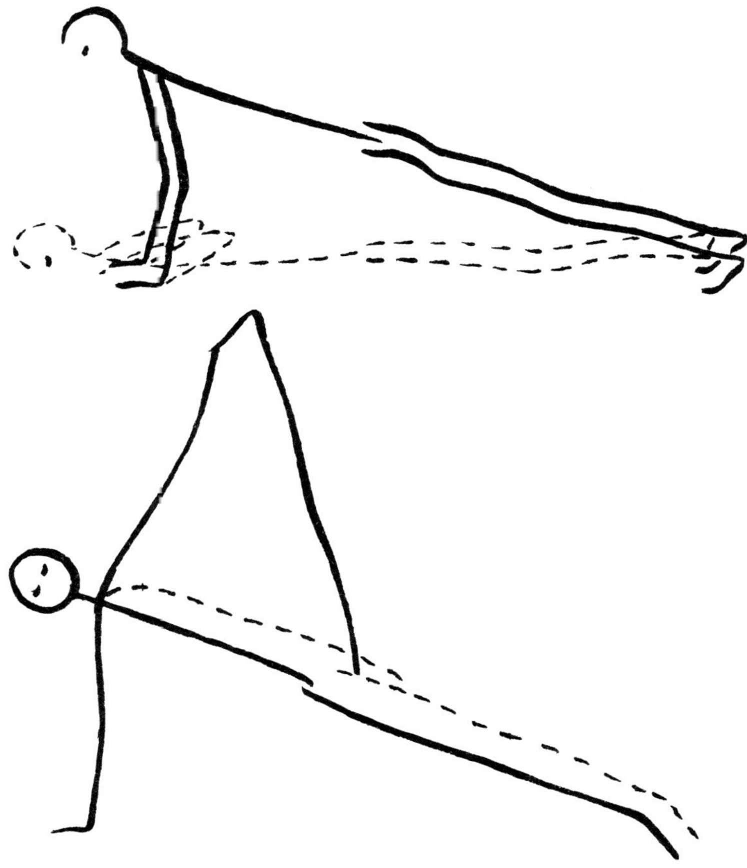

EXERCISE XIV

1. Lie on floor face downward. Hands under armpits, fingers pointed forward. Toes tucked under. (Dotted lines)

2. Raise body off floor by straightening arms. Keep body stiff as a board.

3. With body raised from floor, shift weight of body on to right hand and outside of right foot. Rest left arm over left side of the trunk. Left leg rests on right leg. Keep body straight. Hold. (Dotted lines)

4. Return to starting position and repeat, shifting weight to left side.

5. Then balance on right side again. Bend left leg. Left hand holds on to big toe of left foot and stretches the leg up. Hold.

6. Lower left leg and return to starting position. Shift weight to left side and raise right leg.

EXERCISE XV

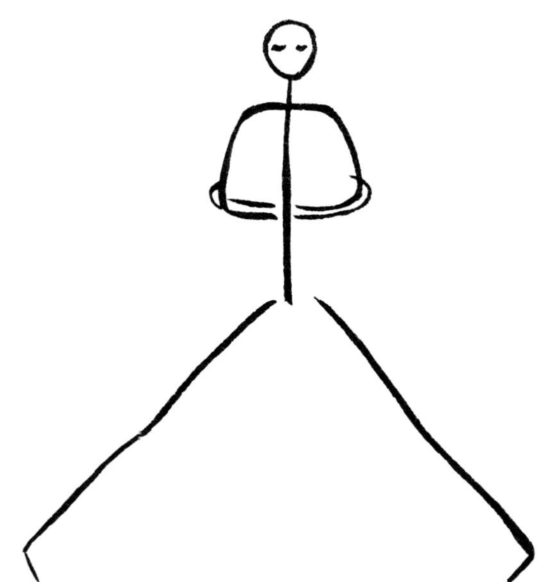

1. Stand with feet four to five feet apart. Arms behind back. Hold on to elbows.

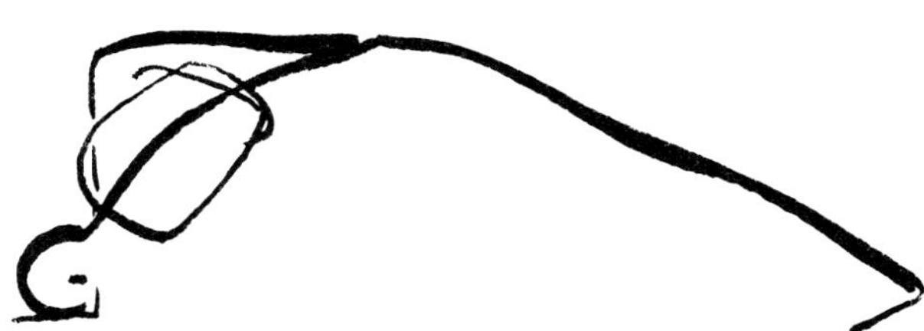

2. Turn both feet to the right. Head, trunk, and pelvis face to the right as well. Bend right leg and move head forward toward right foot. Right shoulder moves downward on inside of right knee. Forehead tries to touch right foot. Back foot remains flat on floor. Come up. Repeat on other side.

3. Hamstring and Leg Muscles

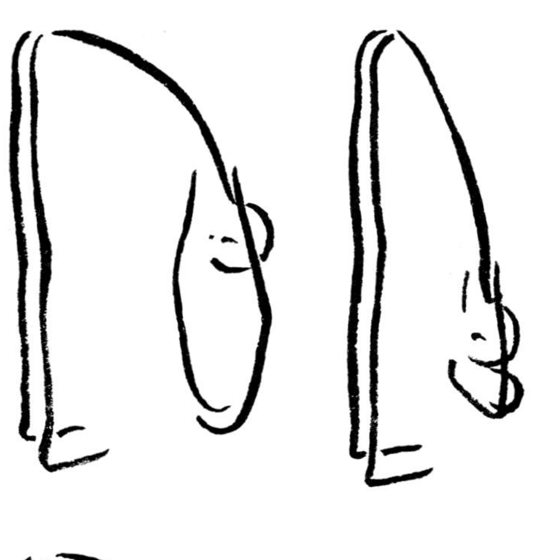

EXERCISE XVI

1. Stand with feet two to three inches apart. Toes pointed forward. Hang forward from the hips, keeping legs straight. Drop arms. If fingers touch floor, then fold arms. Relax neck, shoulders, spine, diaphragm, and stomach muscles. Hang on as long as comfortable.

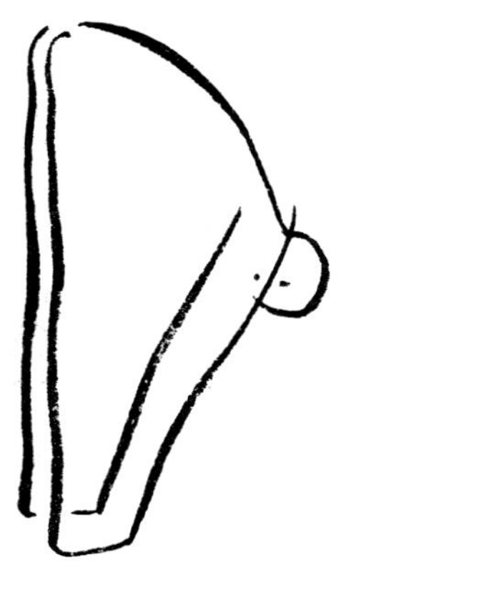

2. Hold on to the back of the knees, calves, ankles, or hook the index and middle fingers round big toes. (See drawing p. 29.)

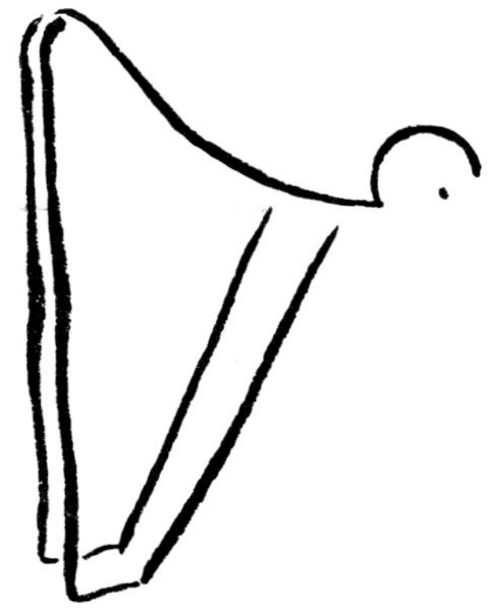

3. Then, hollow the spine and stretch chestbone forward. Look up.

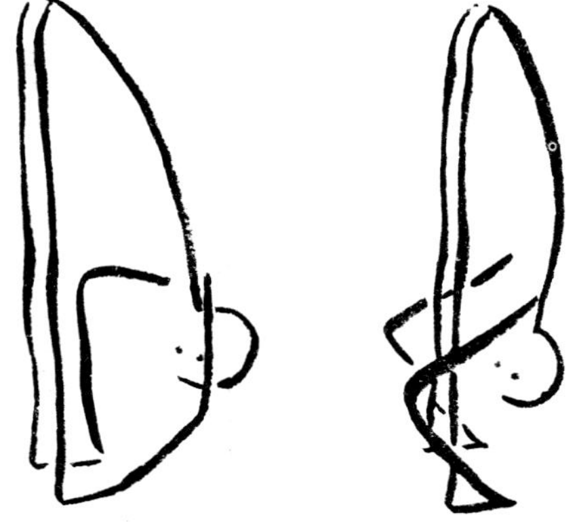

4. Bend elbows toward floor and gently pull chestbone toward knees. Hips and tailbone move upward, ribs move downward. Keep diaphragm and stomach muscles relaxed. Stretch the spine.

EXERCISE XVII

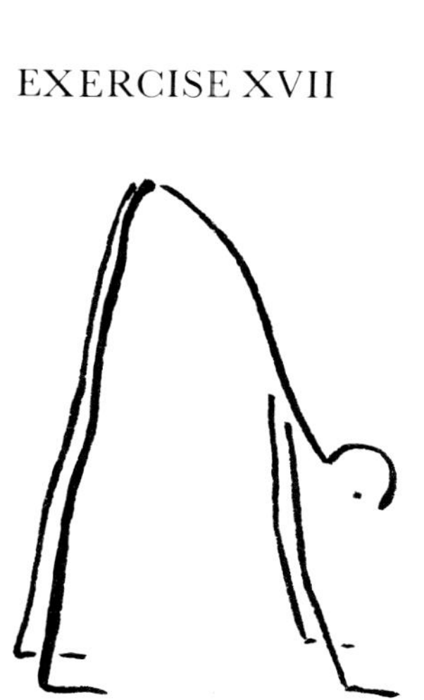

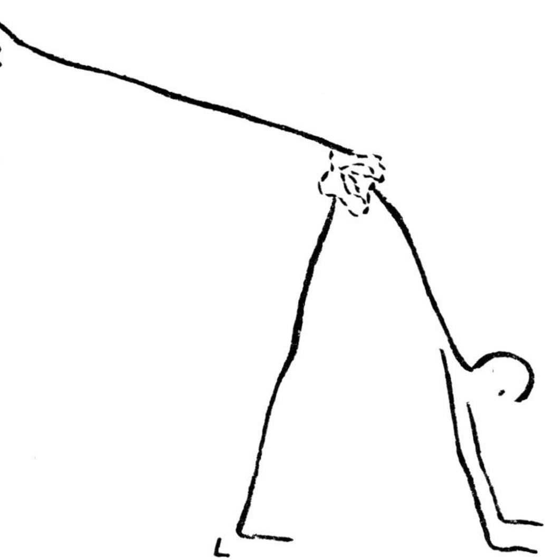

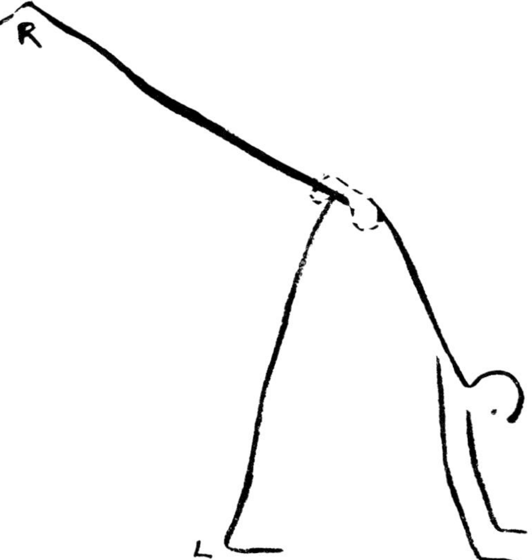

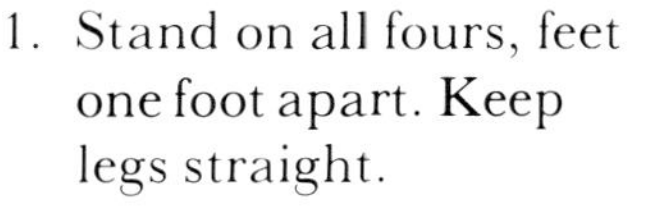

1. Stand on all fours, feet one foot apart. Keep legs straight.
2. Stretch right leg upward and backward. Move right hipbone upward, so that pelvis faces wall to your right side.
3. Then move pelvis down, so that it comes to horizontal position. Keep stretching leg upward. Repeat many times. Return to starting position.

   Repeat on other side.

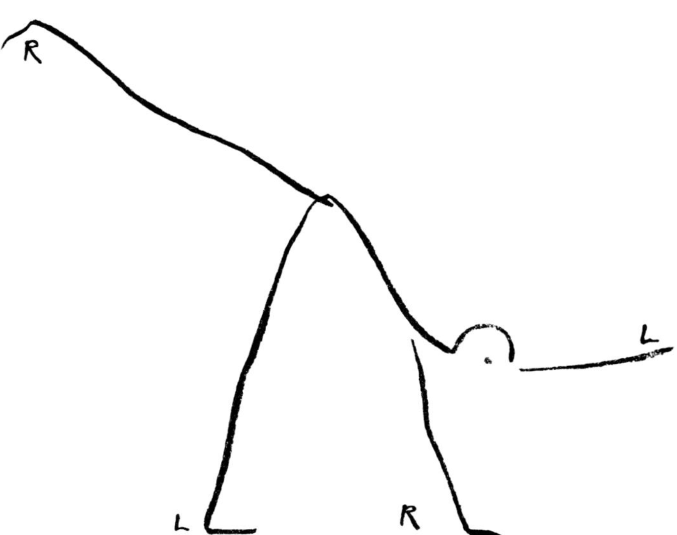

EXERCISE XVIII

Raise right leg again. Raise left arm upward and forward. Hollow the spine. Look up. Keep left foot flat on floor. Bring leg and arm back down.

Repeat on other side.

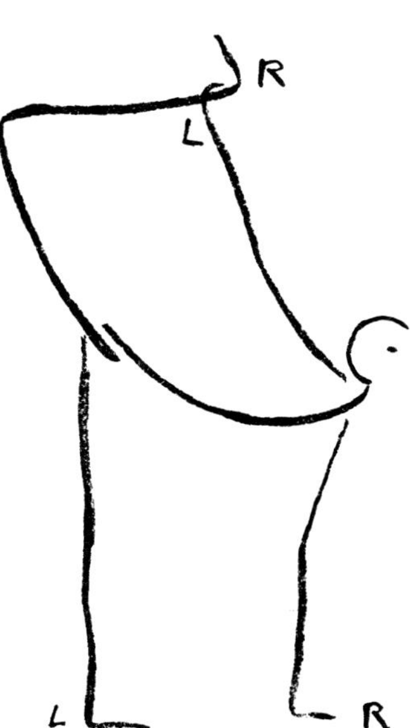

EXERCISE XIX

Again raise right leg. Bend knee. Hold right foot or ankle with left hand. Keep left leg straight. Hollow spine. Look up. Move right foot upward, away from the buttocks. Hold. Come back on all fours.

Repeat on other side.

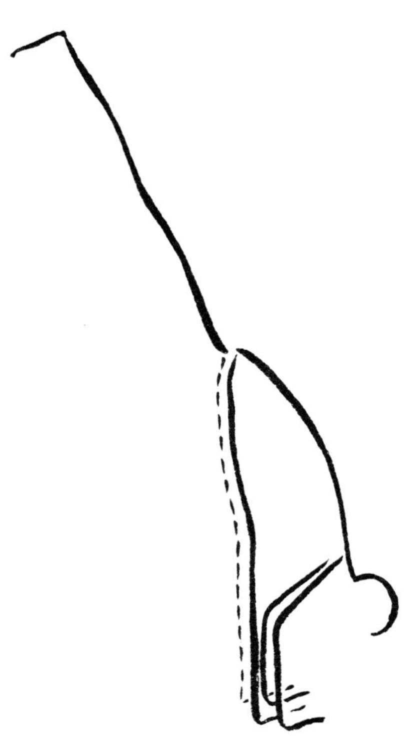

EXERCISE XX

1. Stand with feet a foot apart, toes pointed forward. Hang forward. Place palms flat on floor on either side of left foot. Fingers point forward. Raise right leg upward and backward. Flex heel. Chin moves toward shin bone.

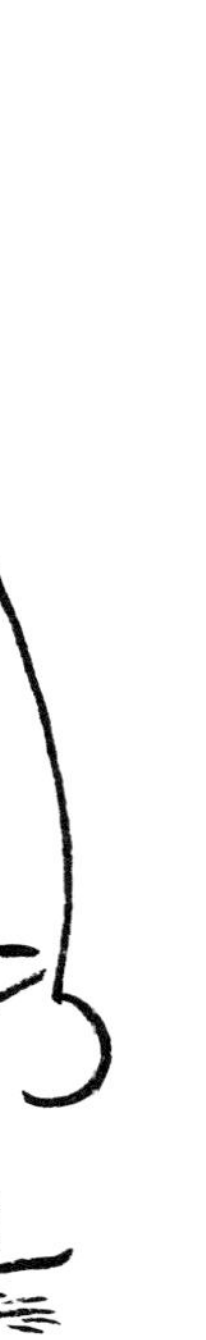

2. Then hold on to left ankle with right hand. Increase forward bend by gently pulling chin closer to leg. Raise right leg further upward. Bring leg back down.
Repeat with other leg.

EXERCISE XXI

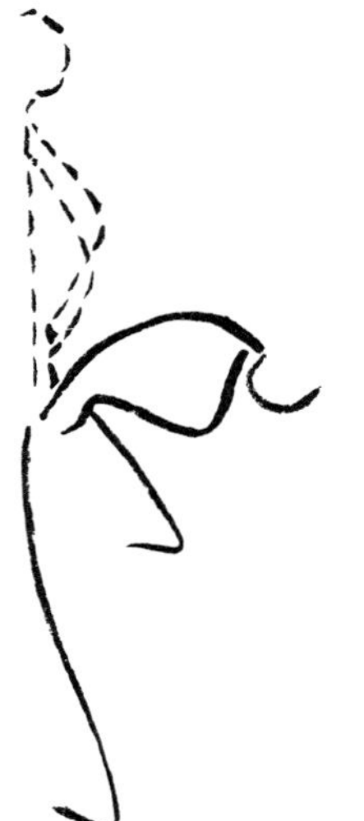

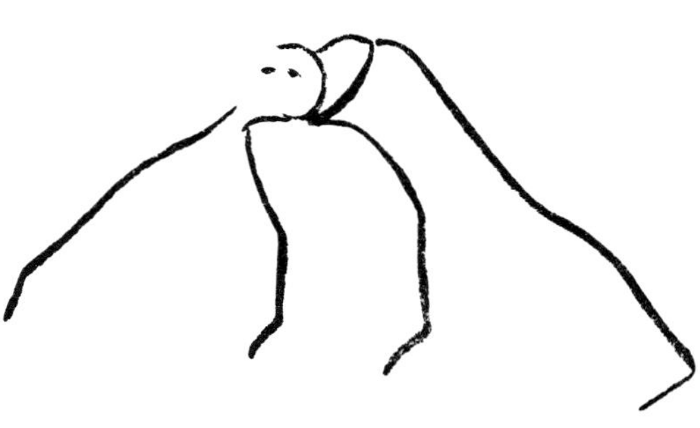

1. Stand with feet as wide apart as possible. Make sure feet cannot slip. Legs straight, toes pointed forward. Hands on back of hips. Arch spine and hang backward. Relax neck, drop head, and look at wall behind you. Push pubic bone forward. Come up.
2. Then bend forward and place both hands on floor between feet. Fingers pointing forward, hands in line with shoulders. Knees straight. Dig palms into floor and look up. Hollow spine, stretch chestbone forward, and move tailbone upward.
3. Bend elbows backward and place top of head on the floor. Hold. Come up. Repeat many times.

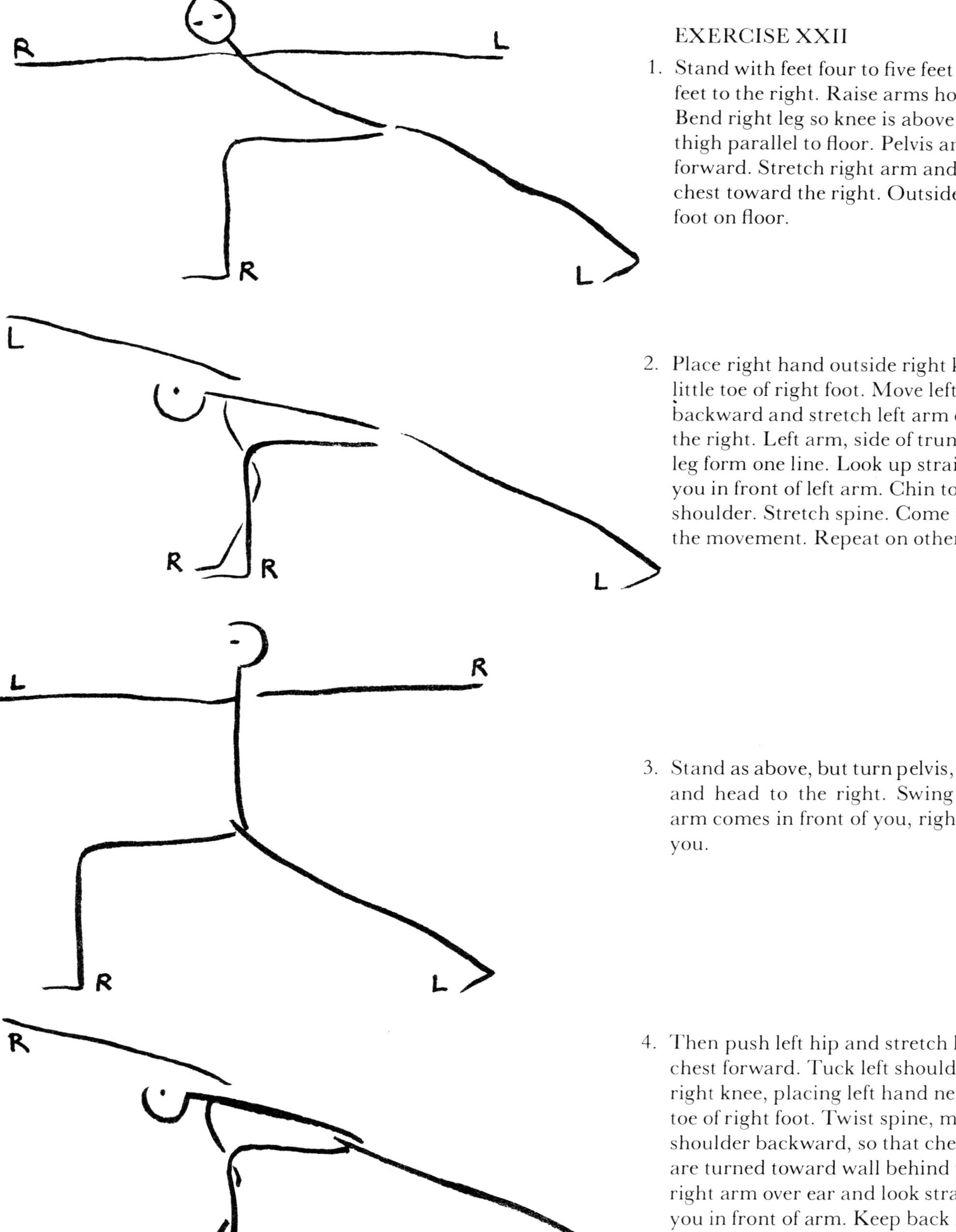

EXERCISE XXII

1. Stand with feet four to five feet apart. Turn feet to the right. Raise arms horizontally. Bend right leg so knee is above heel and thigh parallel to floor. Pelvis and chest face forward. Stretch right arm and right side of chest toward the right. Outside edge of left foot on floor.

2. Place right hand outside right knee next to little toe of right foot. Move left shoulder backward and stretch left arm over ear to the right. Left arm, side of trunk, and left leg form one line. Look up straight above you in front of left arm. Chin toward the shoulder. Stretch spine. Come up reversing the movement. Repeat on other side.

3. Stand as above, but turn pelvis, chest, and head to the right. Swing arms so left arm comes in front of you, right arm behind you.

4. Then push left hip and stretch left side of chest forward. Tuck left shoulder outside of right knee, placing left hand next to little toe of right foot. Twist spine, moving right shoulder backward, so that chest and face are turned toward wall behind you. Stretch right arm over ear and look straight above you in front of arm. Keep back leg straight, outer edge of foot on floor.

   Repeat on other side.

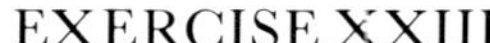

EXERCISE XXIII

1. Stand with feet two to three feet apart. Turn both feet to the right. Raise arms horizontally. Open chest. Relax shoulders. Pelvis and chest face forward. Push tailbone forward. Move right hand to your right, stretching right side of chest. (Dotted lines)

2. While stretching, bend so that right hand touches leg or reaches floor next to little toe. Stretch left arm upward and look past thumb. Tuck chin in. Stretch spine from tailbone to base of skull. Keep moving left hipbone backward and tailbone forward. Right foot and shoulders in straight line. Avoid swinging forward. This is the triangle position.
   Repeat with other arm and leg, turning feet to left.

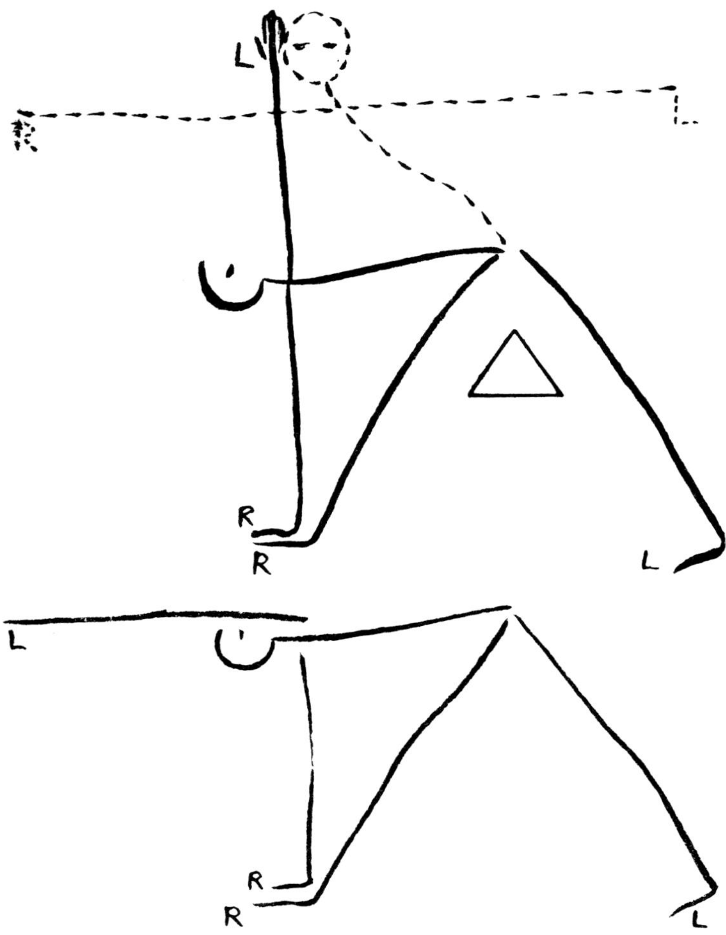

3. Now, in triangle position, move left arm over ear to the right. Shoulder moves backward, arm straight and horizontal, palm down. Look upward in front of you.
   Repeat with other arm and leg.

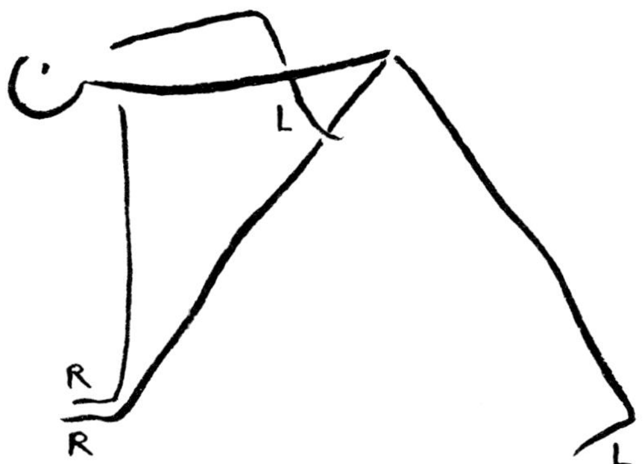

4. Then bring left arm behind back. Tuck fingers in front of right thigh. Pull left shoulder further backward. Keep looking upward.
   Repeat with other arm and leg.

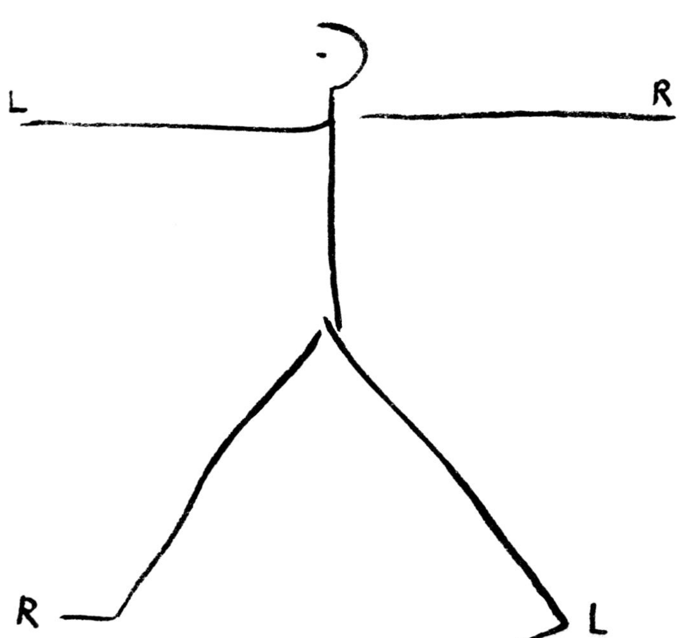

EXERCISE XXIV

Begin as in top drawing; but turn hips, chest, and head to the right, so that left arm comes forward and right arm backward. Push left hip forward.

Then stretch left side of chest, bending forward from hips until spine and arm are in a horizontal position. Place left hand on right leg or next to little toe of foot. Stretch right arm up and look past thumb of right hand. Dig left heel firmly into ground, keeping leg straight. Move right hip backward. Chest faces as much as possible wall behind you. (Solid lines in top drawing show correct position, except that now the arms are reversed and the left hip should move forward rather than back.)

Repeat on other side.

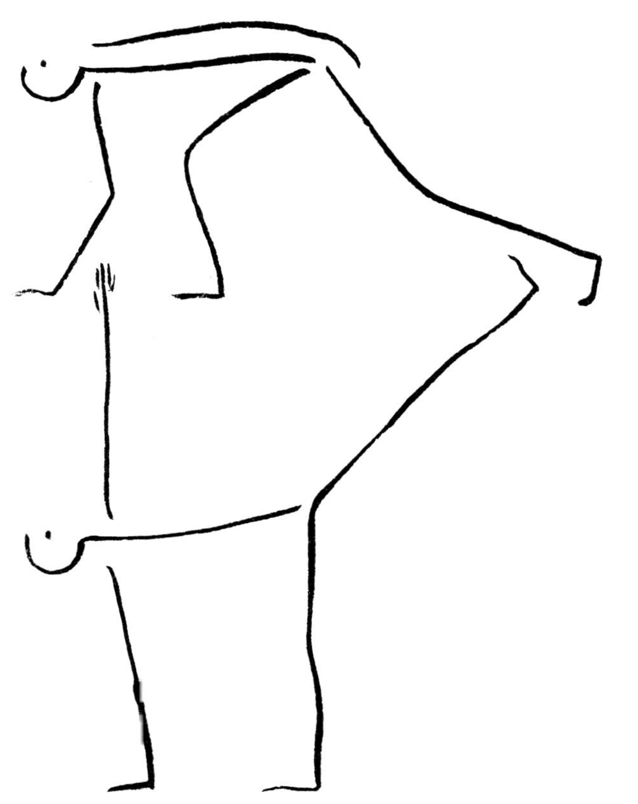

EXERCISE XXV

1. Stand in triangle position. Bend right leg. Place right hand one foot away from right foot on the floor, fingers pointing to the right. Rest left hand over side of left hip.

2. Shift weight of body on to right leg and arm. Straighten right leg and raise left leg. Move left hipbone upward, so that pelvis faces forward. Move left shoulder backward, so that chest and shoulders face forward. Look at wall in front of you. Then stretch left arm up and look past thumb of left hand. Balance and hold.

3. Then bring left arm behind back, tuck fingers over front of right thigh, and pull left shoulder further backward (as in third drawing, p. 40.) Look up.
   Repeat on other side.

EXERCISE XXVI

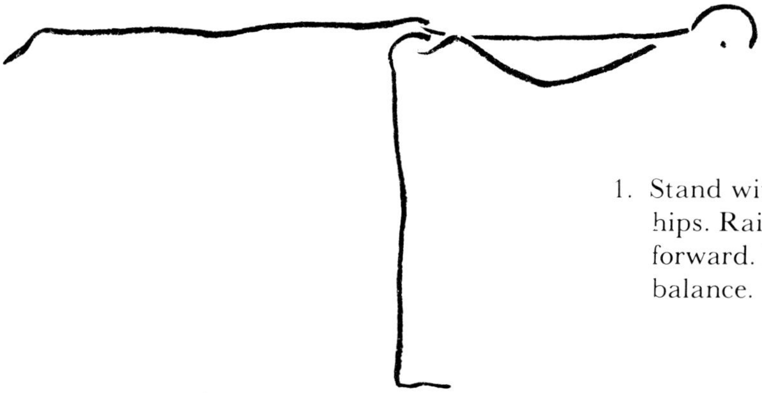

1. Stand with feet slightly apart, toes pointing forward, hands on hips. Raise left leg backward, keeping it straight. Lean trunk forward. Raised leg and trunk are parallel to floor. Maintain balance.

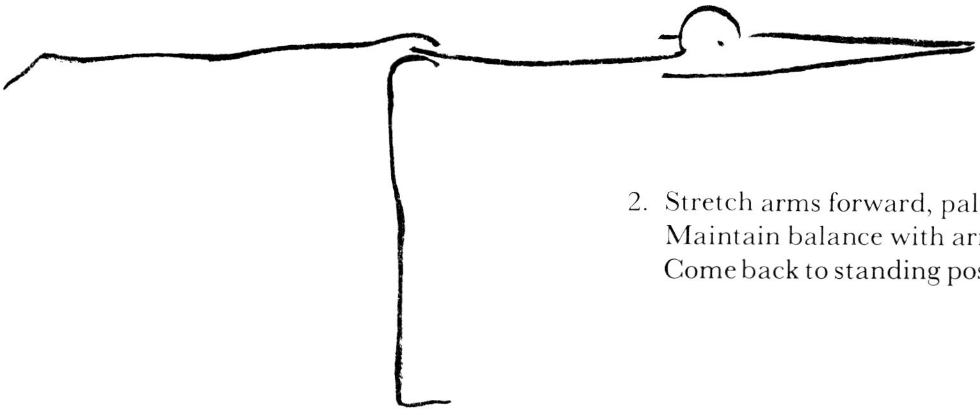

2. Stretch arms forward, palms together, thumbs locked. Maintain balance with arms, back, and leg parallel to floor. Come back to standing posture and repeat with other leg.

EXERCISE XXVII: WARRIOR POSITION

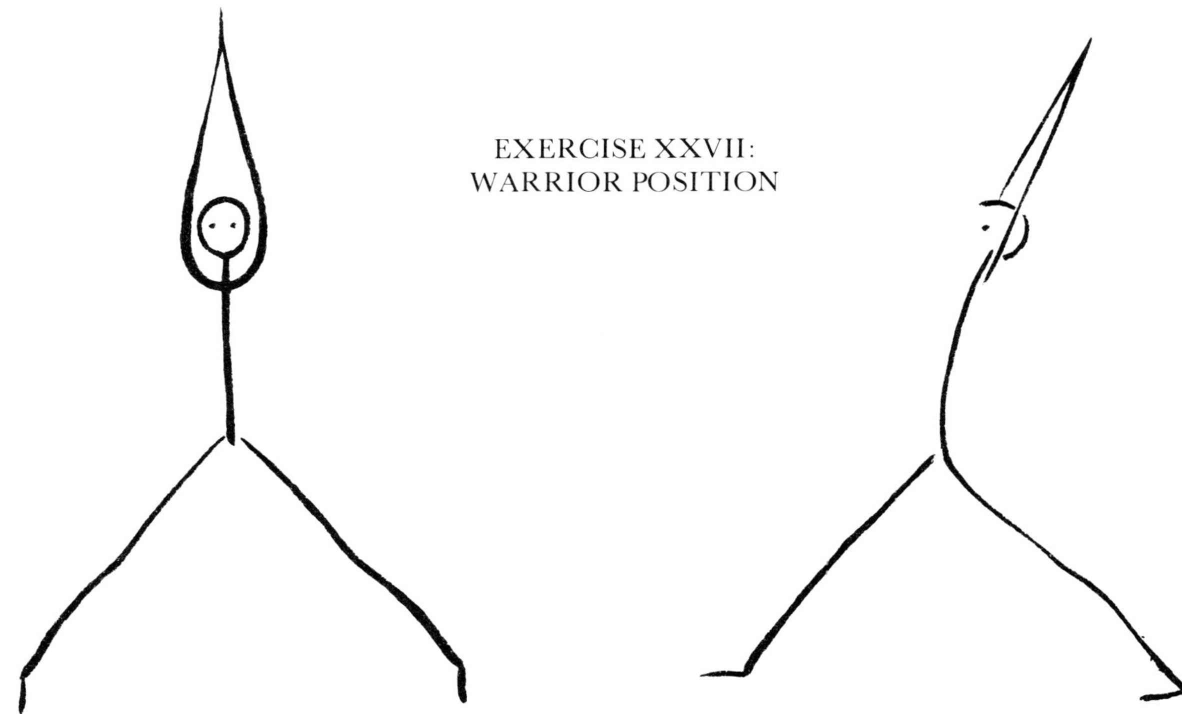

1. Stand with feet four to five feet apart. Stretch arms up and bring palms together. Lock thumbs. Keep elbows straight.

2. Turn feet to right. Face, shoulders, and pelvis face to right. Arms stretch up, elbows behind ears. Spine straight. Push left hip and shoulder forward. Legs straight.

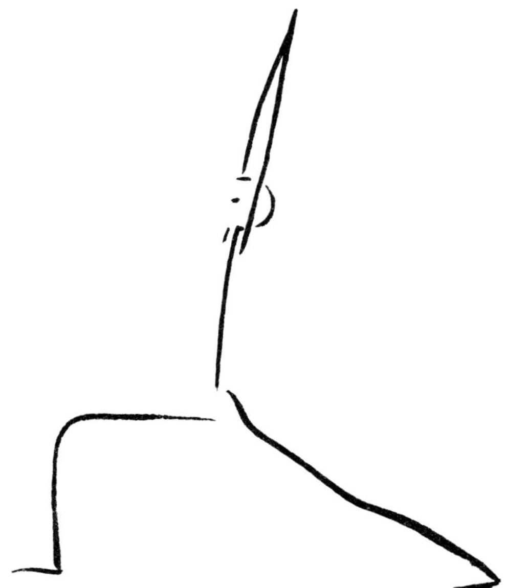

3. Bend right leg, so that knee is straight above heel and thigh comes parallel to floor. Back heel remains on floor.

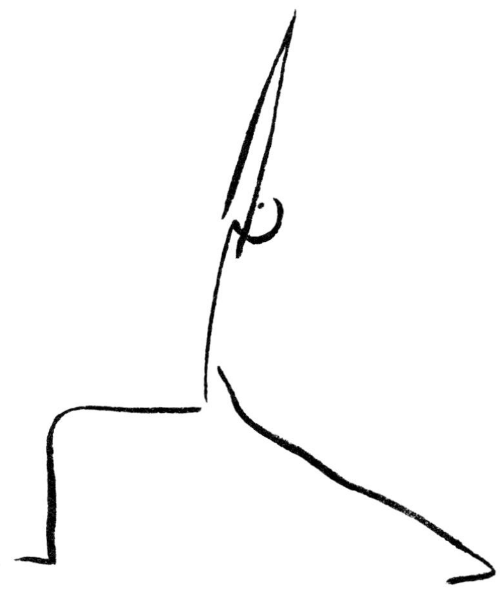

4. Drop head backward and look up at ceiling. Maintain posture. Repeat with other leg.

3. Hamstring and Leg Muscles

EXERCISE XXVIII

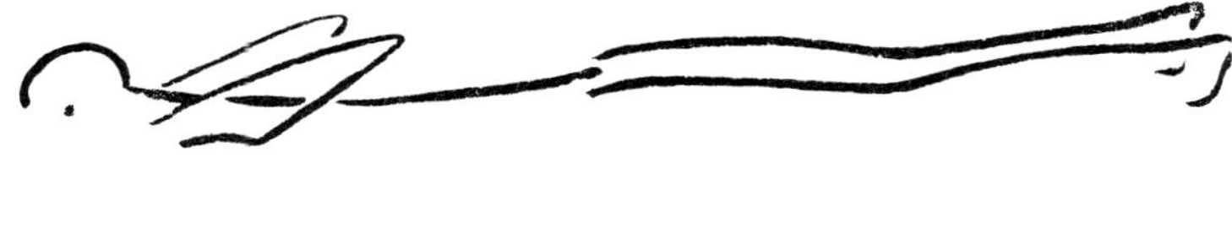

1. Lie on floor face downward. Place hands under armpits. Fingers pointed forward, behind armpits. Elbows back. Toes tucked under.

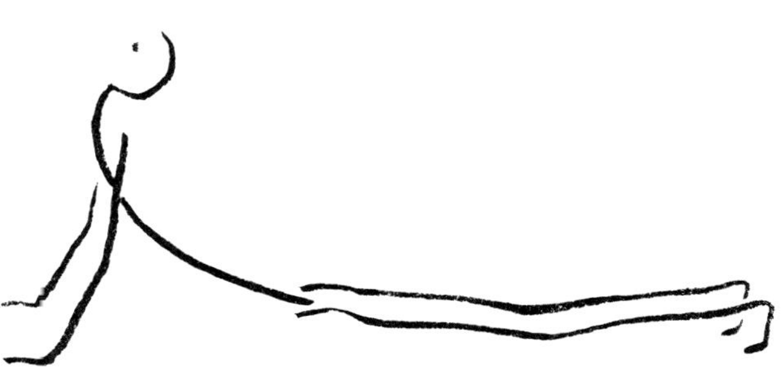

2. Lift body off floor and come up standing on hands and feet. Straighten arms. Push heels backward and down towards floor. Move buttocks and tailbone upward. Arch spine. Push chest and armpits towards floor. Relax neck and drop head towards the floor. This is the dog position.

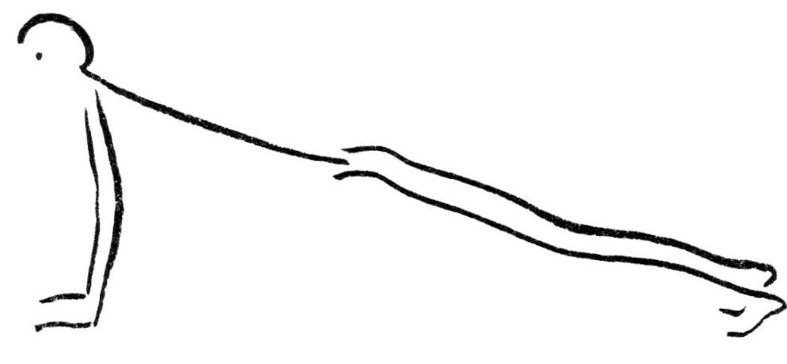

3. Then lower pelvis until it hangs two inches above floor. Hollow spine. Look upward. Hang comfortably in this position.

4. Then lift pelvis and straighten body. Make it stiff as a board. From heels to shoulder is one straight line. Arms straight.

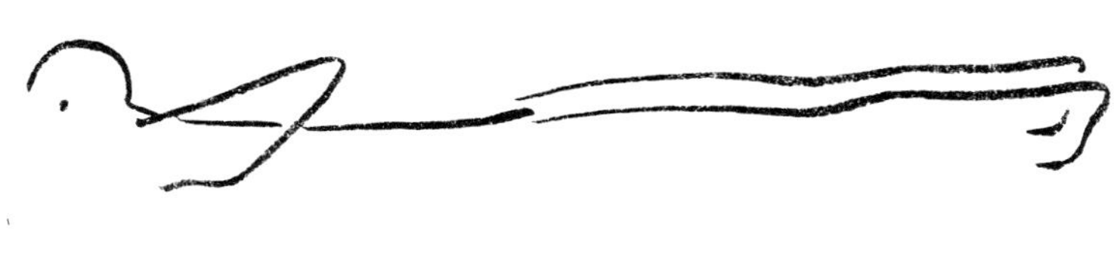

5. Bend elbows backward, lowering body until it is suspended in a straight line two inches above floor. Head, chest, stomach, pelvis, and legs do not contact the floor.

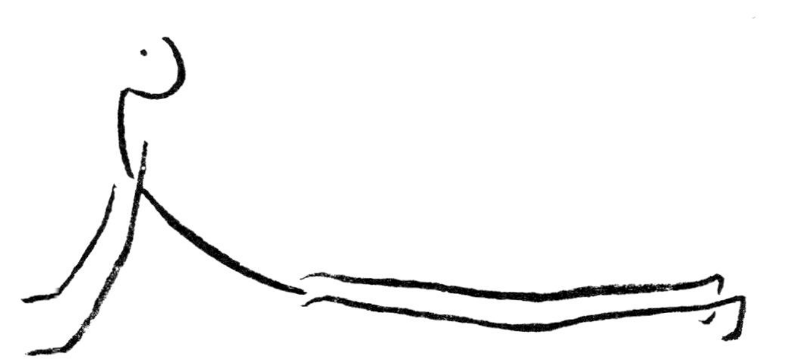

6. Then straighten arms, hollow the spine, and look upward.
   Then swing pelvis up and backward to return to dog position (2).
   Repeat whole cycle many times.

4. KNEES

The knee is the largest joint in the body. It must sustain great stress, as it is located between the hip and ankle joints, supporting the entire weight of the body above the knee. But the knee is not simply a fixed pillar of strength; it must have freedom of motion for walking. The knee is principally a hinge joint with basic functions of flexion and extension. However, some of its ligaments are constructed in an unusual fan-shaped pattern so as to allow a certain looseness when the knee is in a flexed position; this is especially important when walking or running. Again, consider that sitting regularly on the floor will increase the flexibility and strength of the knee.

EXERCISE I

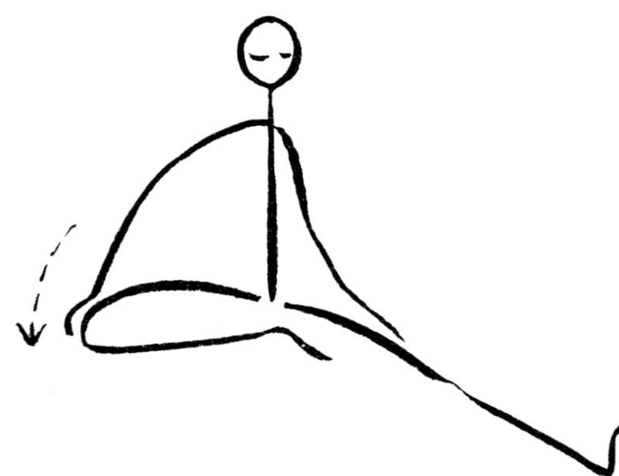

1. Sit on floor. Place sole of right foot against inside of left thigh. Keep left leg straight. With right hand bounce knee downward to touch floor.

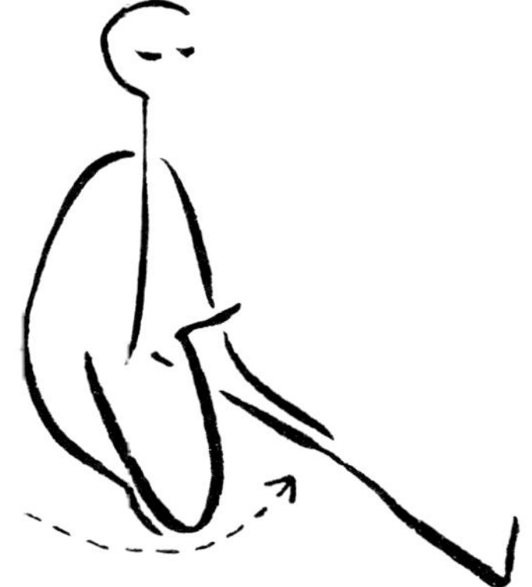

2. Place right ankle as high up as possible on thigh or in left groin. Keep left leg straight, toes pointing upward. With right hand bounce knee downward and toward left knee. Right knee will eventually touch floor next to left knee.

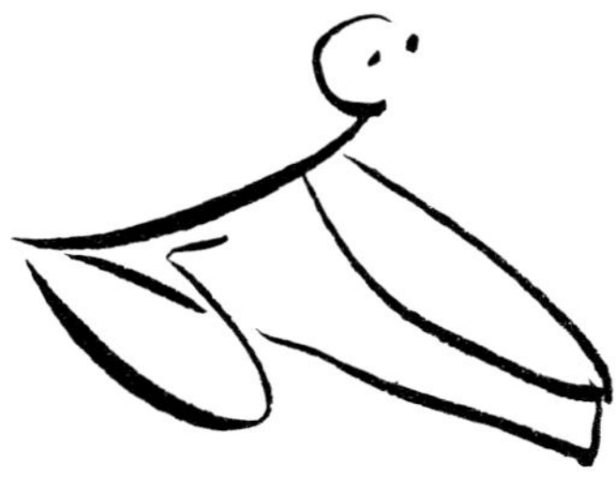

3. Keeping right ankle in position, hold left knee, calf, or foot with both hands. Hollow spine. Look up.

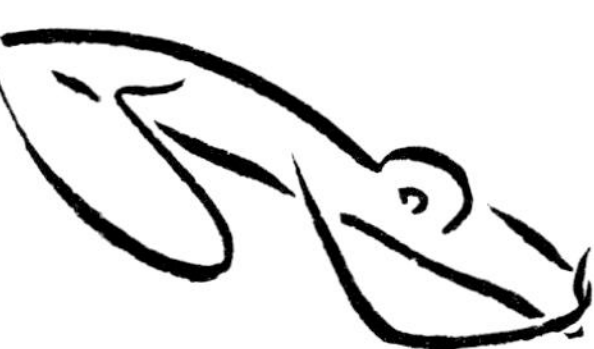

4. Then pull chestbone toward left knee. Elbows bend and stretch forward. Relax and hold. In this position heel of right foot will eventually push into left side of lower abdomen.
Repeat on other side.

EXERCISE II

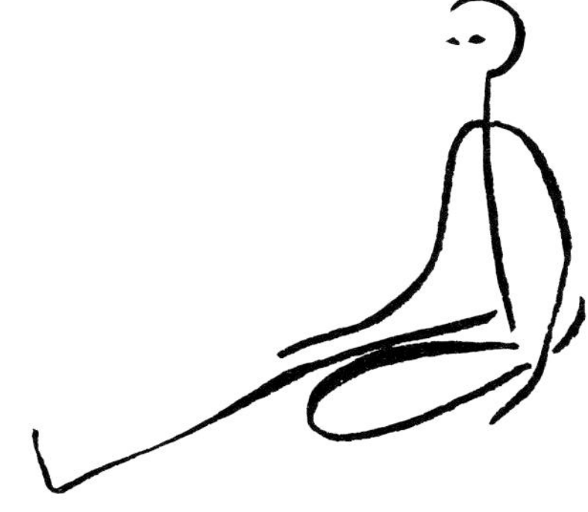

1. Sit on floor. Place left foot next to left buttock; left knee next to right knee. Front of foot and ankle rest on floor, sole of foot faces upward, big toe in contact with left buttock. Keep right leg straight. Both buttocks on floor.

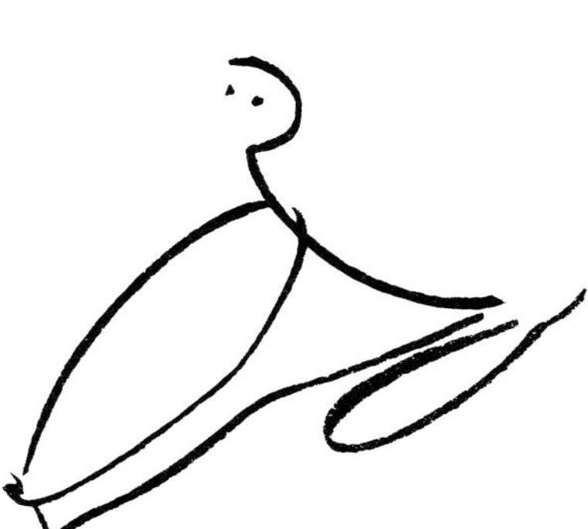

2. Hold right leg or foot with both hands. Arch spine. Look up.

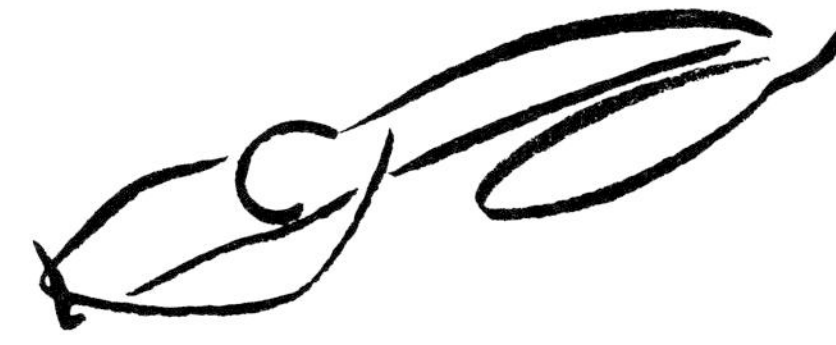

3. Pull chestbone forward toward knees. Relax and hold.

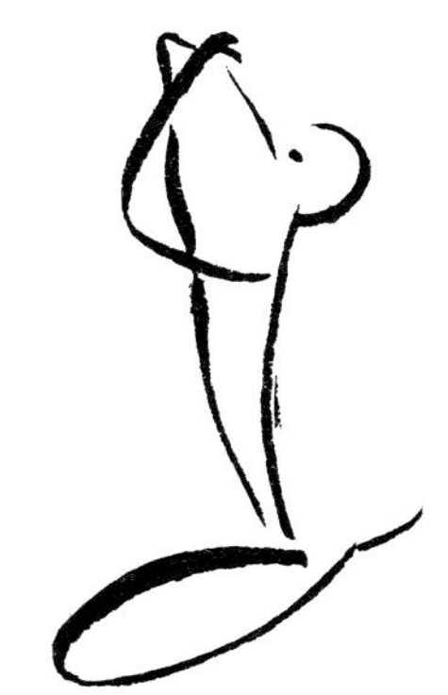

4. Return to position 1. Then pull right knee toward chest. Hold right foot with both hands. Stretch right leg upward. Keep spine straight. Hold and relax.
   Repeat with other leg.

EXERCISE III

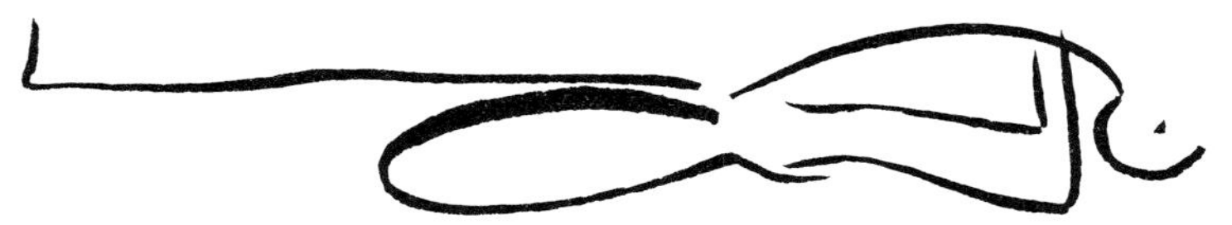

1. Sit on floor, left foot next to and curling round left buttock. Knees together. Both buttocks on floor. Lean back on elbows. Arch spine and neck. Place top of head on floor.

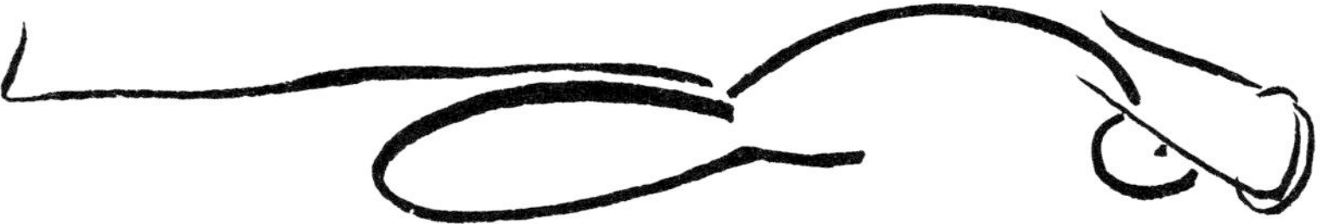

2. Bring arms over head toward floor. As arms relax, elbows will sink down to floor.

3. Now lie down so back contacts floor. Knees together. Stretch arms above head. Hold and relax.

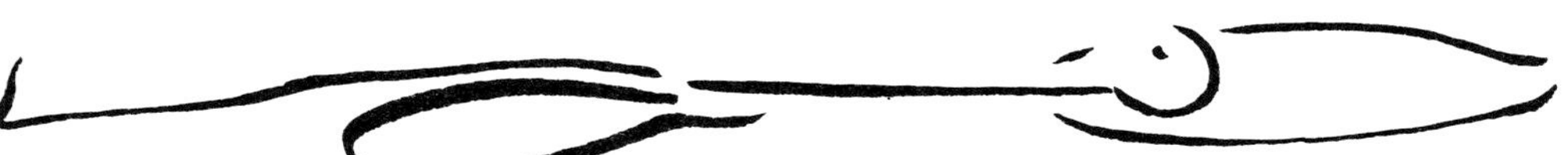

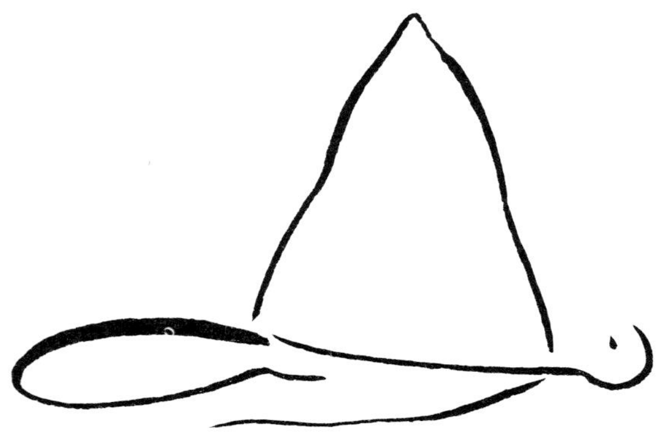

4. Bring arms down. Pull right knee toward chest. Right hand holds right foot or leg. Stretch leg upward. Left knee remains on floor.
Repeat exercise with other leg.

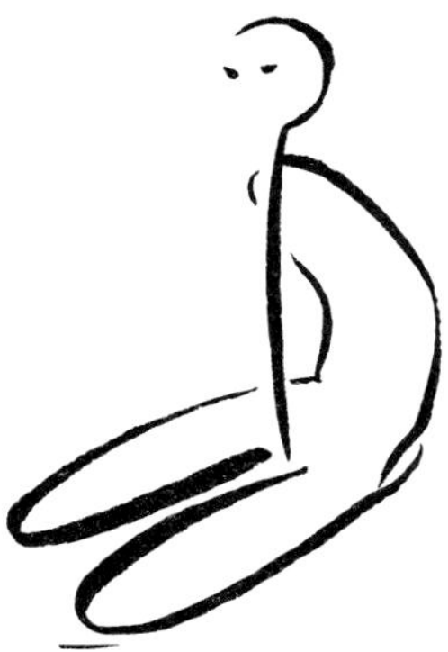

EXERCISE IV

1. Sit on floor. Bend legs at knees and place feet outside and next to buttocks. Push calf muscles outward, so that thickness of calves does not prevent legs from bending. Knees together. Hold on to toes.

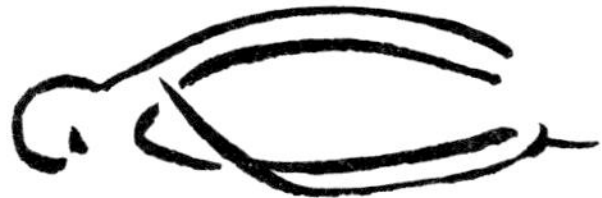

2. Bend forward, resting chestbone on thighs, forehead on floor. Try to keep buttocks on floor. Relax spine. Hold.

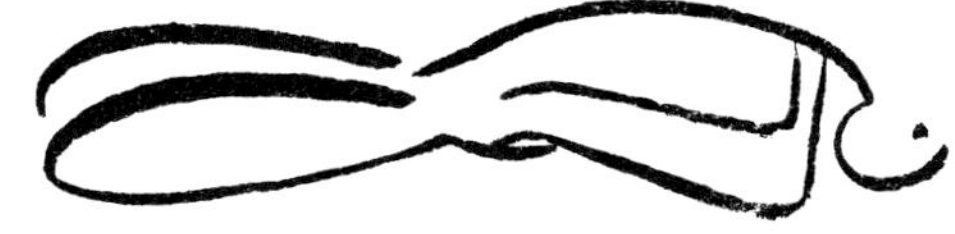

3. Then lean backward on elbows. Arch spine and neck. Keep knees together.

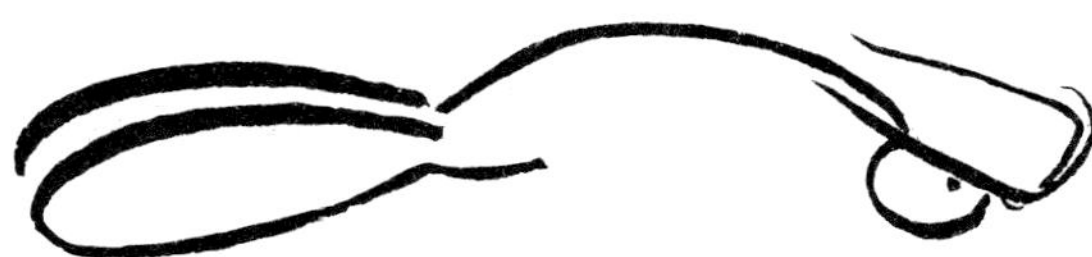

4. Put top of head on floor. Bring arms over head toward floor. Hold elbows. Relax. Elbows will sink down toward floor.

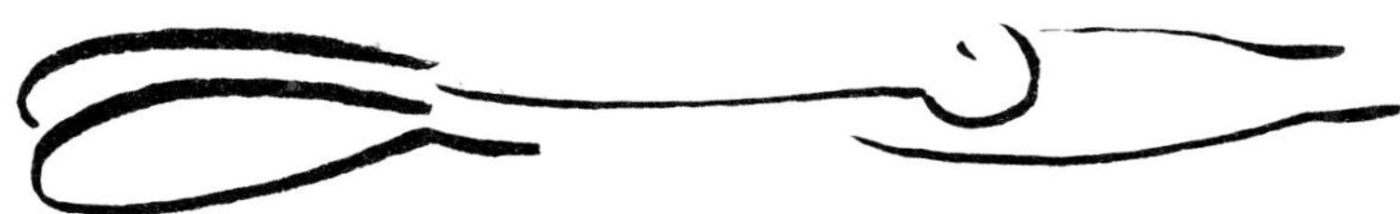

5. Now lie down, so that entire back touches floor. Stretch arms over head. Relax and hold.

The deep thigh muscles pull on the five lumbar vertebrae. When these muscles are sufficiently stretched, entire spine will contact floor.

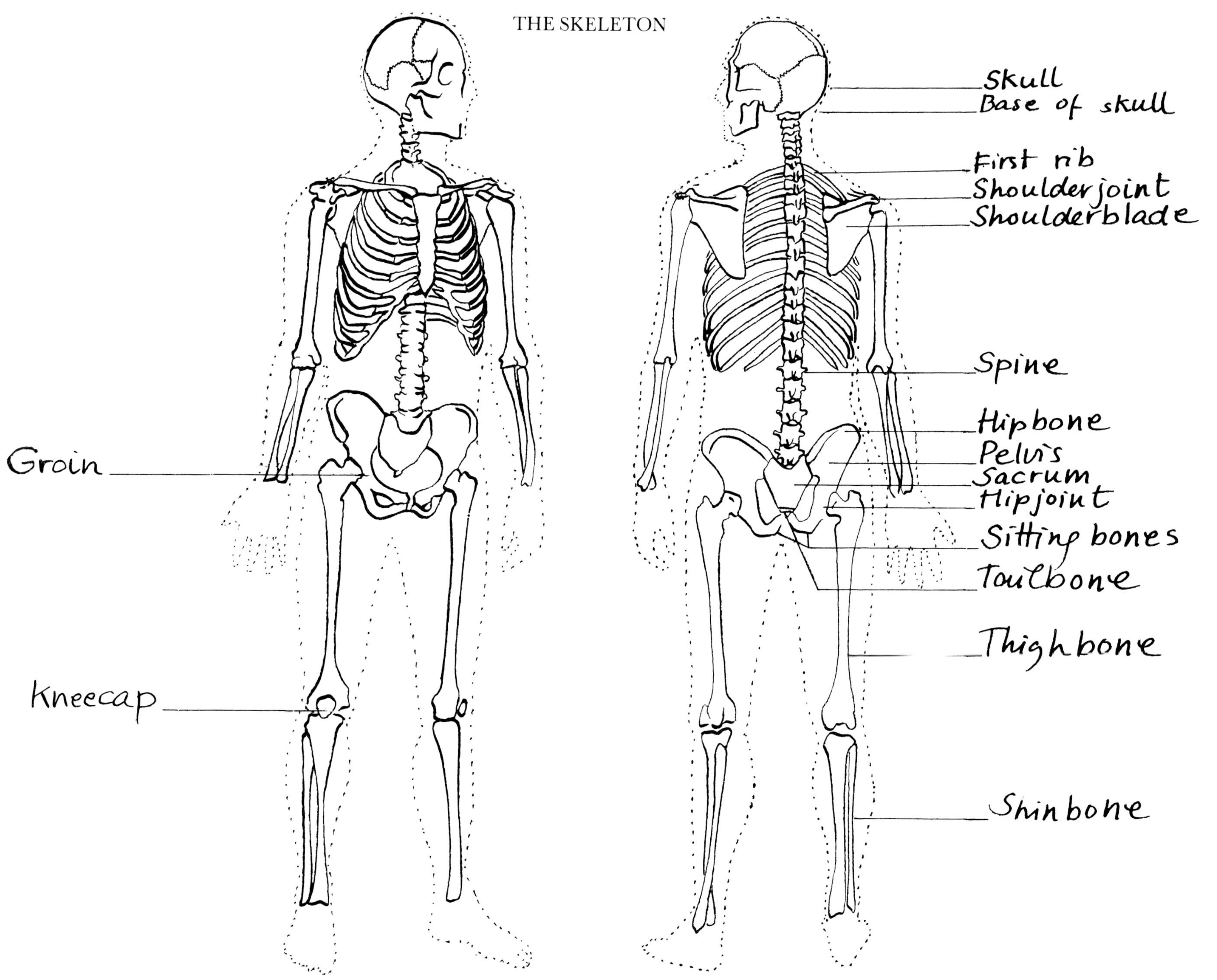
Skull
Base of skull
First rib
Shoulderjoint
Shoulderblade
Spine
Hipbone
Pelvis
Sacrum
Hipjoint
Sitting bones
Tailbone
Thighbone
Shinbone
Groin
Kneecap

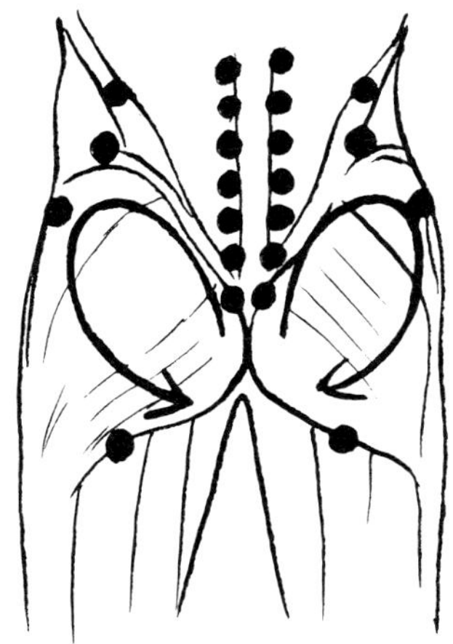

5. PELVIS, HIPS AND BUTTOCKS

How much time do you spend each day sitting in a chair? Besides shortening tendons and hamstring muscles, furniture stiffens the thigh joints and throws the pelvis into an extremely unnatural position. Consider Lewis Carroll's Tweedle-dum and Tweedle-dee: their names are representative of their physical and mental state. From their chestbone down to their knees there is nothing but a balloon of fat. In their dance with Alice they could manage only four turns round the tree before dropping from exhaustion.

Since the middle section of the body is the centre for so many movements of the whole body, it must be loose and flowing. The hip is a ball-and-socket joint, capable of movement in all directions. Stand up and move your legs (one at a time) from the hip in as many ways as possible: forward and backward, side to side, in circles. As you repeat the movements, you will feel a stretching and energising sensation in the hip and pelvis area. A tight and stiff pelvis will definitely hamper the flow of sexual energy. As you perform the pelvic clock and related circular exercises, the pelvis will move with increasing looseness and freedom. The lower back is another area of the body both badly abused and little used. As it is the base of the spine (see p. 64), the health of the lower back (and pelvis) is essential to good posture. Stiffness of the lower back will cause frequent neck and head aches, as the tension is reflected upward via the spine. The five vertebrae of the lower back need to be loosened through stretching exercises and massage of tailbone and sacrum pressure points.

EXERCISE I

Lie down on back. Pull knees up, feet off floor. Move knees around as if describing two circles on the ceiling: one clockwise, the other anti-clockwise. Repeat changing direction of circles.

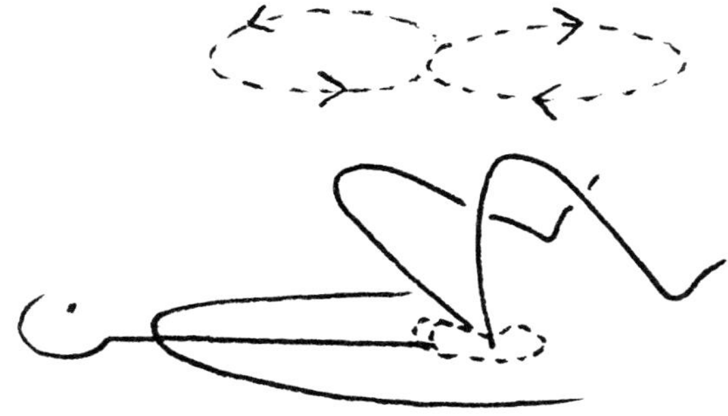

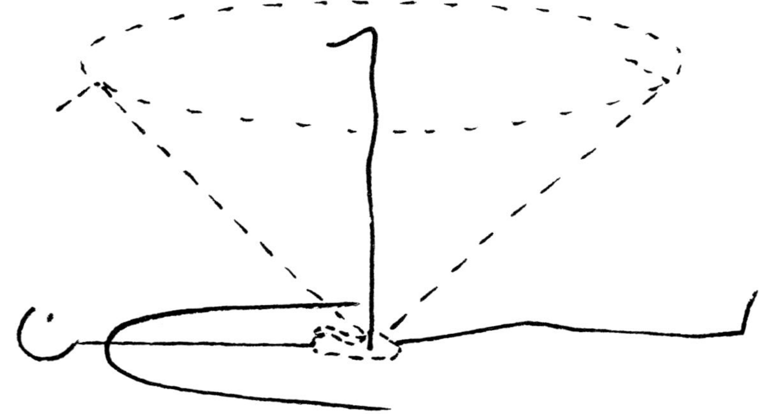

EXERCISE II

Lie down. Stretch right leg upward, heel toward ceiling. Left leg and rest of body relaxed. Turn right leg around in wide circles: clockwise and anti-clockwise. Repeat with left leg.

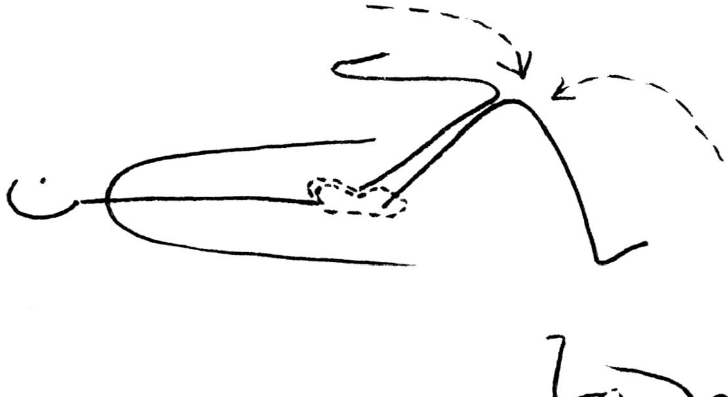

EXERCISE III

1. Lie down. Place feet about one foot away from body. Spread feet until knees drop inward, but do not draw feet towards you. Knees hang above floor but do not touch each other. Gently bounce knees downward. Relax and hold.

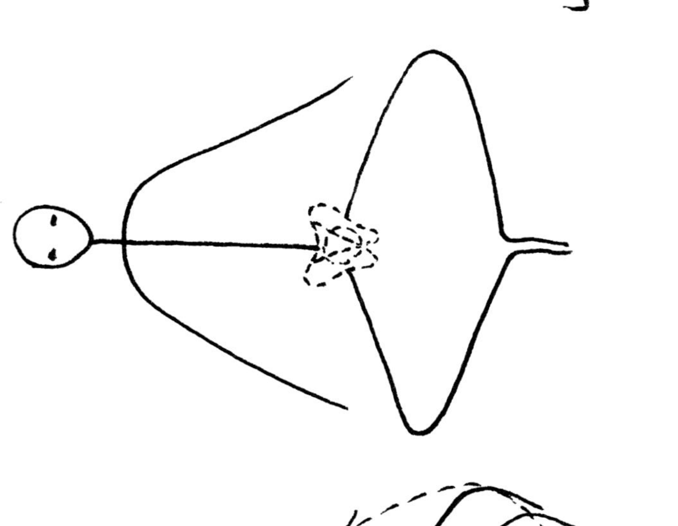

2. Bring soles of feet together. Drop knees outward. Relax and hold.

EXERCISE IV: INDIAN BABY

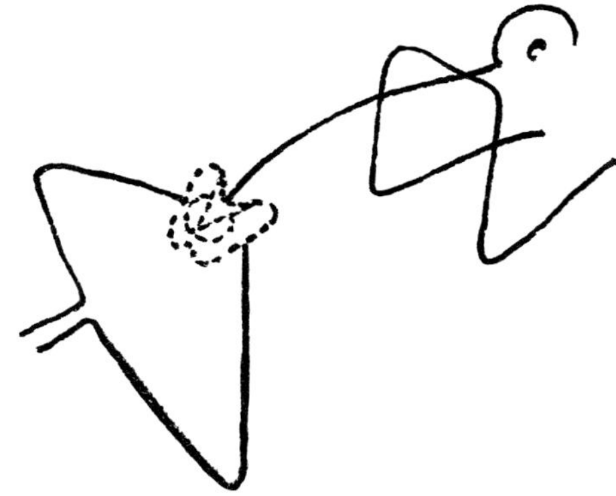

1. Indian babies are carried on the hip by their mothers, and so they have a good, open pelvis and loose hip joints. This exercise helps loosen your hip joints.
   Go down on hands and knees. Place knees as wide apart as possible, soles of feet together. Place hands on floor in front of you and move them slowly foward. Place elbows on floor.

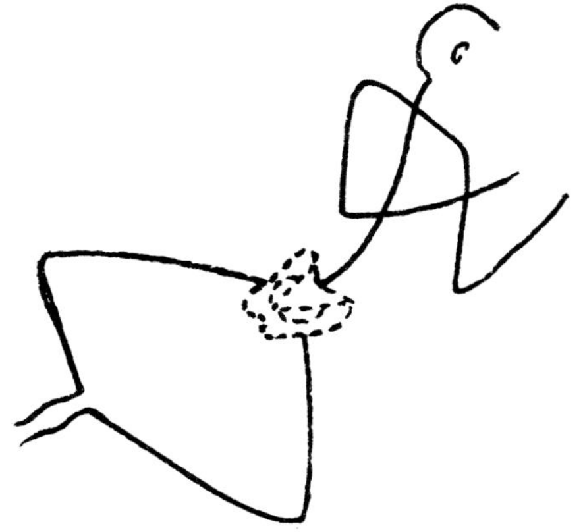

2. Pelvis will sink toward floor. Move hands forward until pubic bone touches floor. Try to keep feet in contact with floor. Relax and hold.

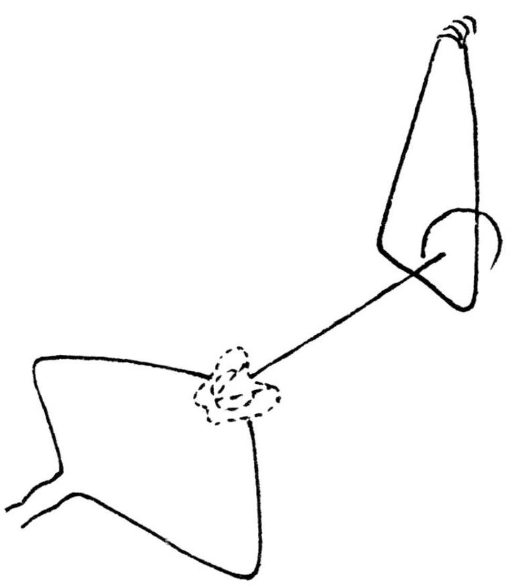

3. Now lie with pelvis, chest, and face in contact with floor. Feet on floor, soles touching. Interlock fingers behind back and stretch hands upward. Arms should make a right angle to floor. Relax and hold.

EXERCISE V

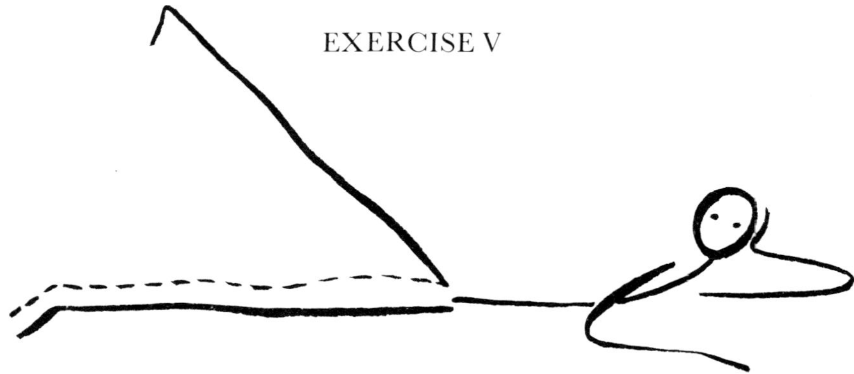

1. Lie on left side. Body and legs form a straight line. Place left elbow on floor, supporting head with left hand. Right hand rests on floor in front of stomach. Raise right leg as high as possible, keeping knee and foot facing forward. Hold. Relax and repeat many times.

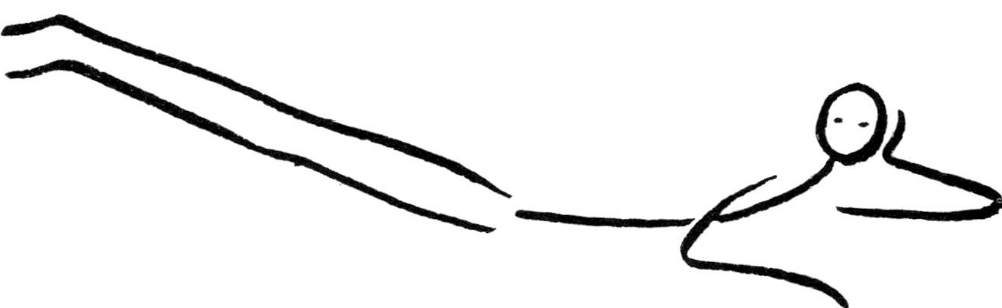

2. Raise both legs off floor as high as possible, keeping legs straight and together. Repeat many times. Repeat exercise on right side.

EXERCISE VI

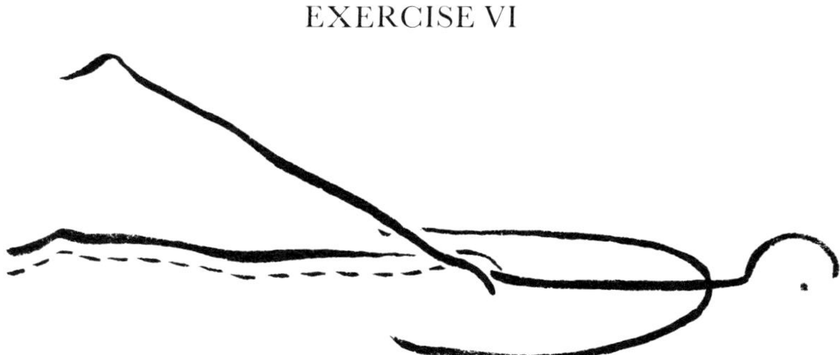

Lie down on stomach, arms relaxed next to body. Raise right leg as high as possible. Keep leg straight. Right hipbone remains on floor. Keep rest of body relaxed.
Lower leg and repeat with left leg.

EXERCISE VII

Lie down on stomach, arms relaxed over head on floor. Raise right leg as high as possible, and in as wide an arch as possible bring it over toward the left. The foot touches floor on left side of body. Right hipbone leaves floor. Keep hands in place. Bring leg back up in arch, and reverse movements. Repeat with other leg.

EXERCISE VIII

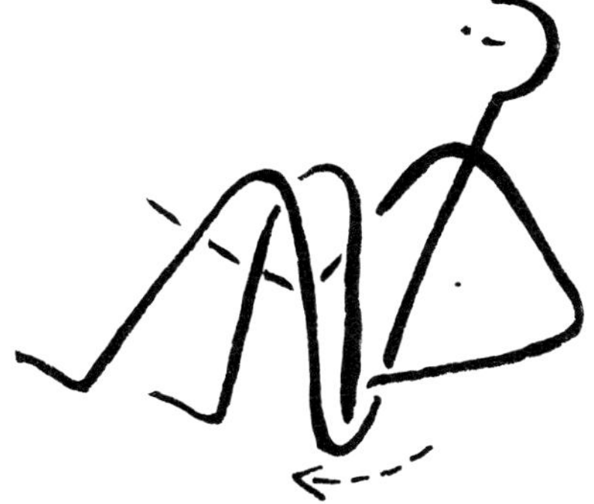

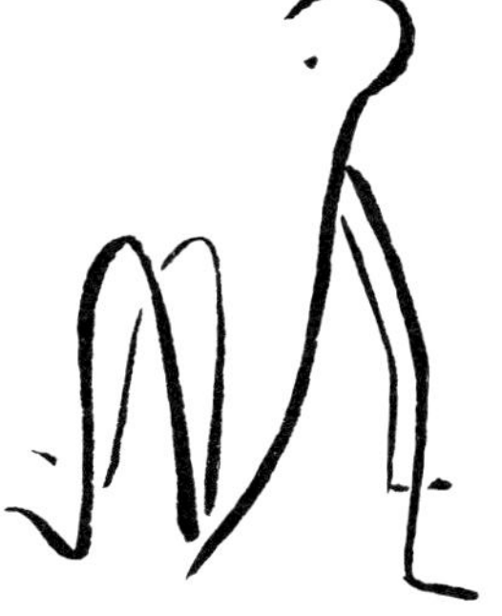

1. Sit on floor. Pull knees toward chest, feet off floor.

2. Lift left buttock off floor and place it one or two inches forward. Then repeat with right buttock. 'Walk' forward around room on buttocks. Then 'walk' backward around room in like fashion.

3. Sit down on floor, hands behind back. Pull knees up so that feet leave floor. Rock pelvis backward so that tailbone contacts floor. Using it as a pivot, rotate pelvis. Massage area around tailbone by rolling it over floor: clockwise and anti-clockwise, slow and fast.

EXERCISE IX: THE PELVIC CLOCK

1. Sit down comfortably, knees apart, soles of feet together. Hands behind body on floor. Imagine you are sitting in the centre of a big clock dial. In front of you is 12; behind you is 6. Rock pelvis forward toward 12; tailbone comes off floor. Rock pelvis backward toward 6; now sitting bones come off floor. Rock pelvis forward and backward until movement is loose and easy.

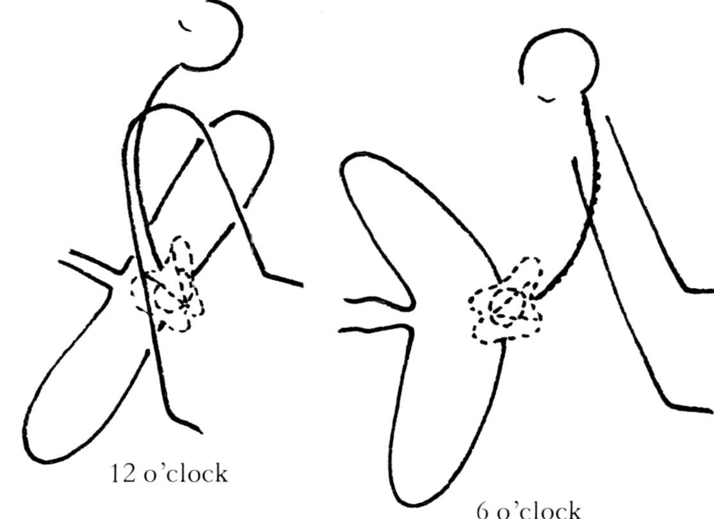

12 o'clock 6 o'clock

2. Rock pelvis to the right toward 3; left buttock comes off floor. Rock pelvis to the left toward 9; right buttock comes off floor. Repeat many times.

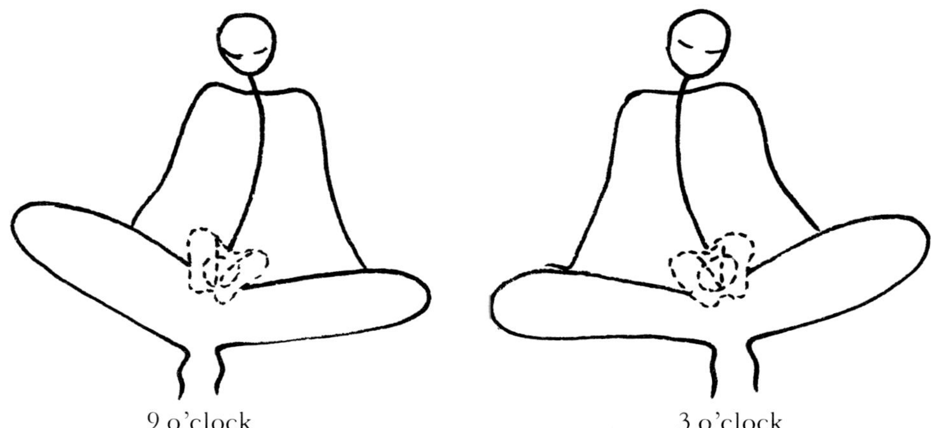

9 o'clock 3 o'clock

3. Rock pelvis to 12. Then move pelvis around clock to 1; then back again to 12. Repeat five times. Then move pelvis from 12 over 1 to 2 and back again. Repeat five times. In like manner move from 12 to 3, 4, 5, and 6, each time returning to 12. Movement should be without any strain. Then lie down, straighten legs, and feel how back contacts floor.
   Come up sitting and repeat same movements on left side of clock.

4. Now move pelvis toward 12 and slowly make a complete circle with pelvis, passing over each digit many times. Slowly increase speed. Repeat many times, clockwise and anti-clockwise. Lie down on back and feel how pelvis contacts floor.

To be fully appreciated, this exercise requires concentration and time. If the exercise has been performed without strain, the lower back should contact or approach quite close to the floor when you lie down.

EXERCISE X

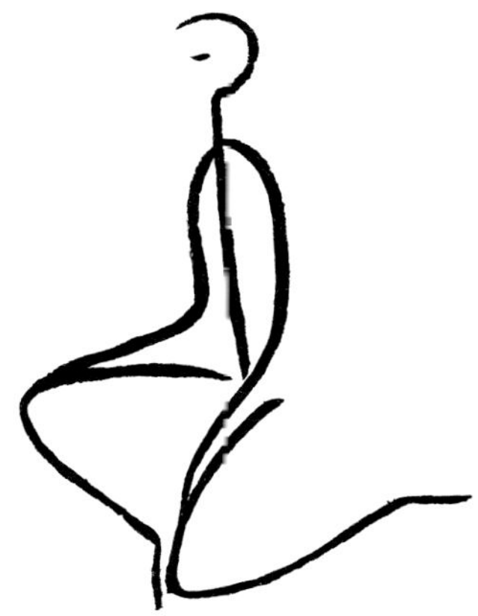

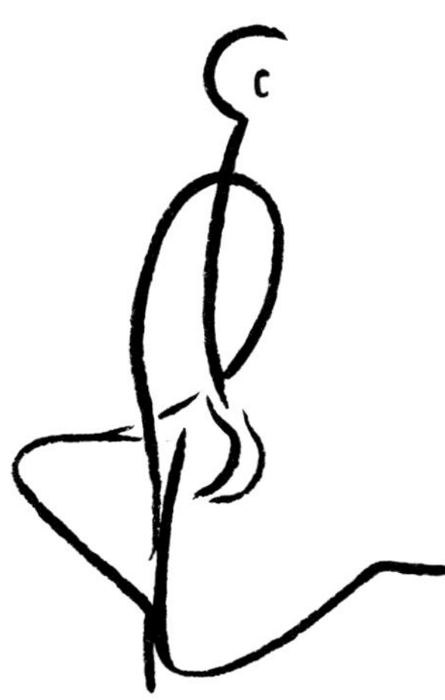

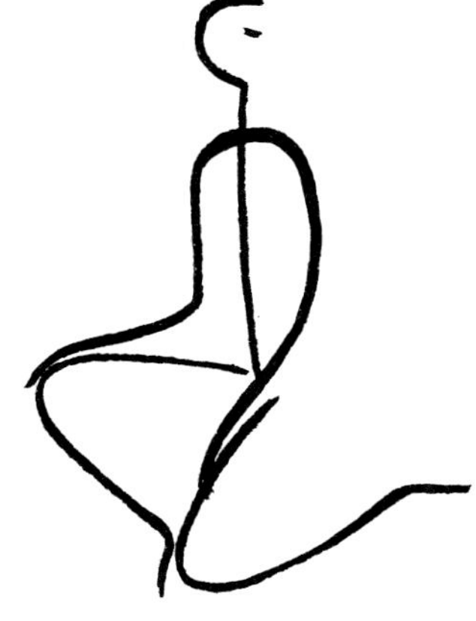

1. Sit on floor. Bend knees and drop them to floor on right side of body. Place sole of right foot on inside of left thigh. Keep both buttocks on floor.
2. Move left hip forward and upward. Left buttock comes off floor. Twist trunk and look over right shoulder to wall behind you.
3. Place left buttock firmly back on floor. Twist trunk to the left. Look back over left shoulder.
Then twist to the right again and raise left buttock.
Repeat many times.
Then repeat dropping legs to the left side.

EXERCISE XI

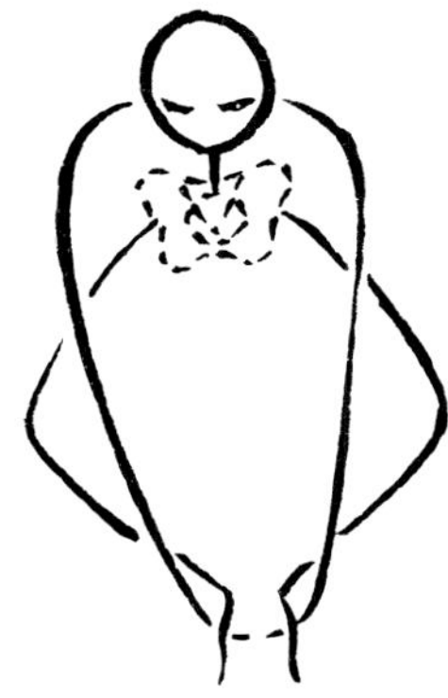

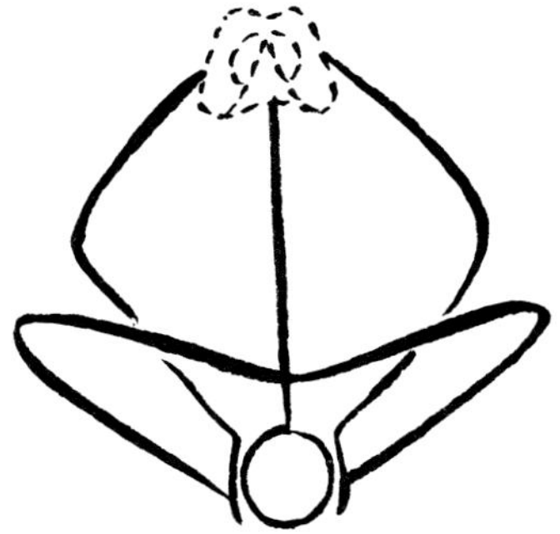

1. Sit down with legs in front of you. Bend knees and drop them outward. Feet should be about one and a half feet away from body and six inches apart with soles facing each other.
Hold on to feet.
2. Bend forward; elbows move outward. Try to place top of head between soles of feet. Relax the back. Hold.

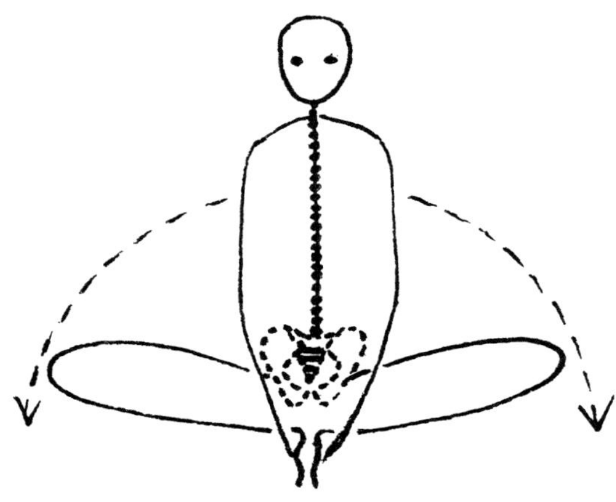

EXERCISE XII

1. Sit on floor on sitting bones, not on tailbone. Bring soles of feet together, heels close to pubic bone. Hands hold feet. Spine straight. This is the tailor position. Bounce knees up and down towards floor. Repeat for at least three minutes.

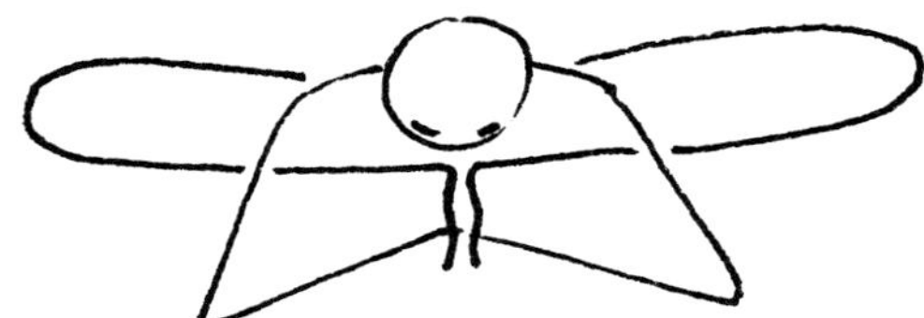

2. Lean forward. Spread elbows and gently bounce them toward floor. Keep spine straight. Chestbone moves forward.

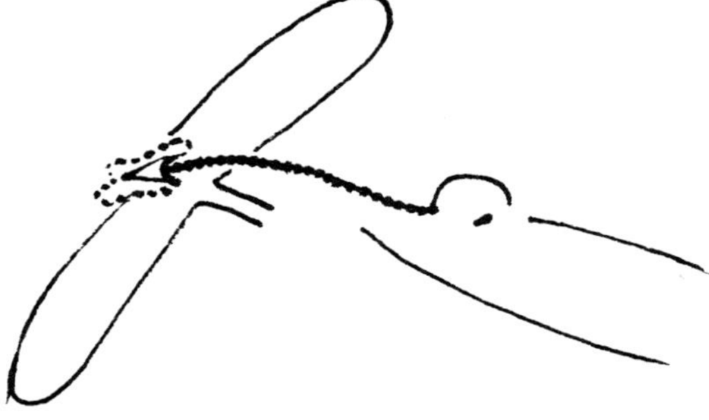

3. Stretch arms forward. Shift weight of body forward. Buttocks come off floor. Balance on outer edges of both feet. Relax and sit down.

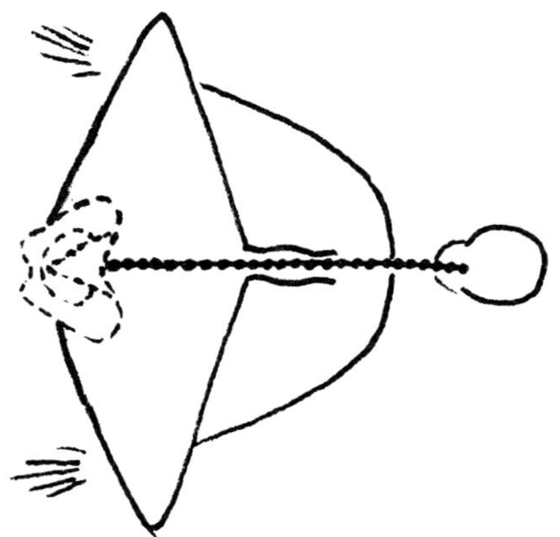

4. Bend forward again, tucking arms under knees. Straighten arms and push top of hands into floor. Lift buttocks off floor. Bounce up and down. Chestbone moves toward feet; chin moves toward floor. Keep soles of feet firmly pressed together.

EXERCISE XIII: HALF AND FULL LOTUS

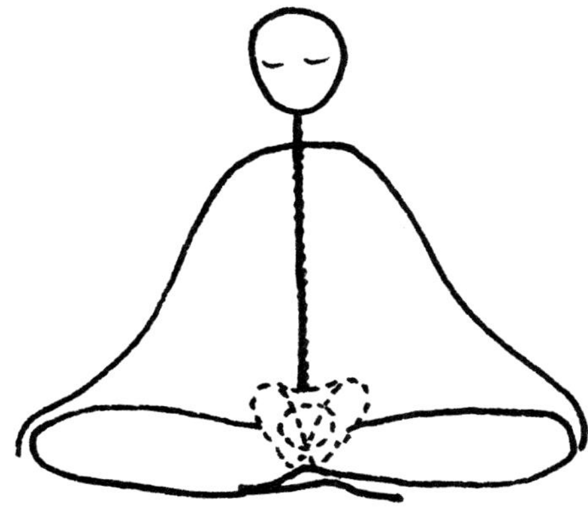

1. Sit on floor in easy position. Bring right heel as close to pubic bone as possible. Bring left foot in front of right foot. Sit on sitting bones, not on tailbone. Spine straight.

2. Pull right foot up on left thigh, as close as possible to left groin. Place left foot underneath right leg. There should be no strain on right ankle. Sit on sitting bones. Spine straight. This is a half lotus.

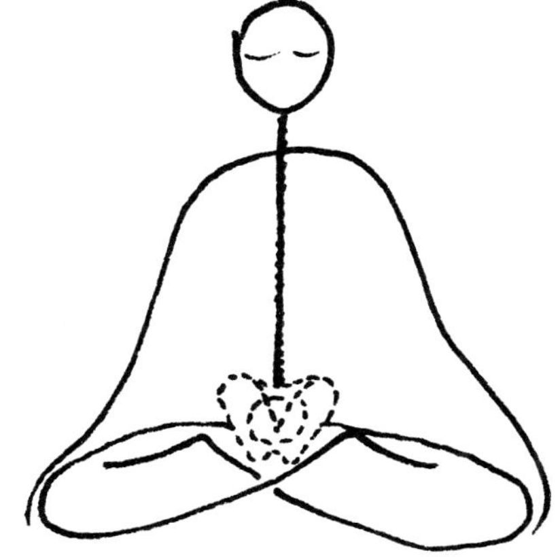

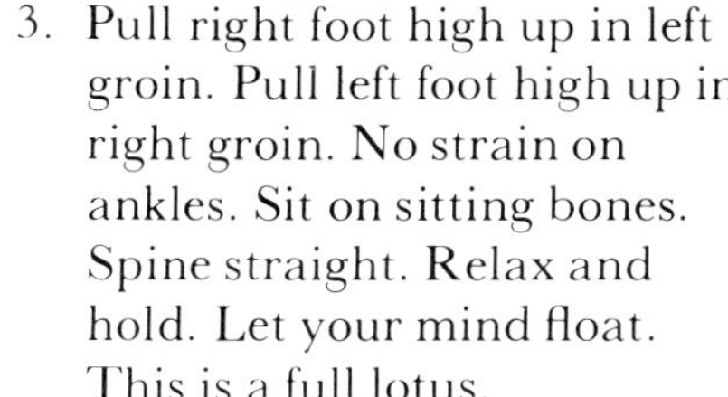

3. Pull right foot high up in left groin. Pull left foot high up in right groin. No strain on ankles. Sit on sitting bones. Spine straight. Relax and hold. Let your mind float. This is a full lotus.

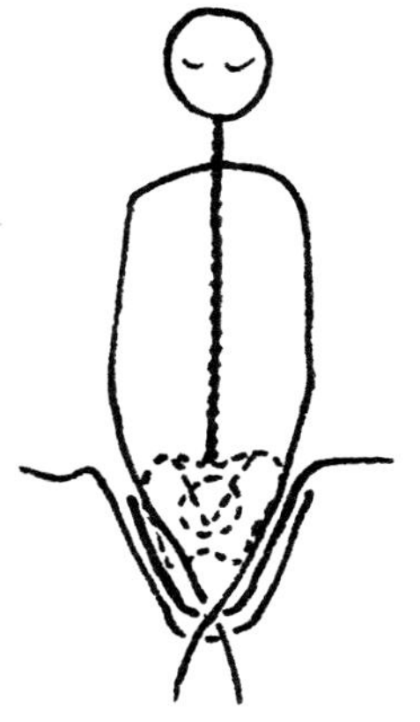

EXERCISE XIV: POSTURE OF PEACE

Sit on floor. Bend right knee and place right heel next to left buttock. Right knee should be directly in front of body. Bring left leg over right leg and bend knee. Left foot rests next to right buttock on floor. Left knee is above right knee. Do not sit on heels. Keep buttocks on floor. Rest right wrist on top of left knee and left wrist on top of right wrist. Spine relaxed.
Relax and hold.

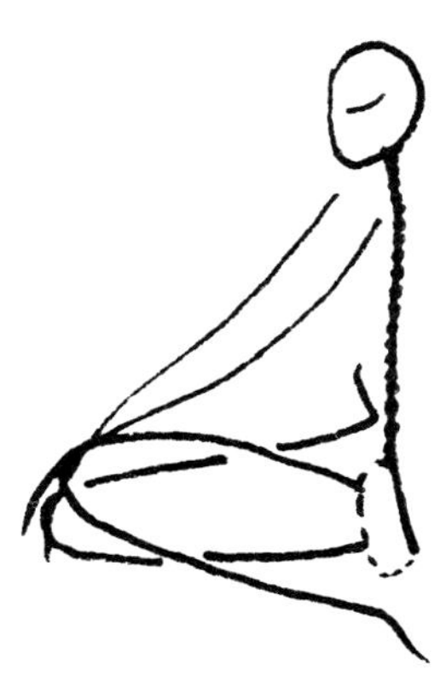

EXERCISE XV

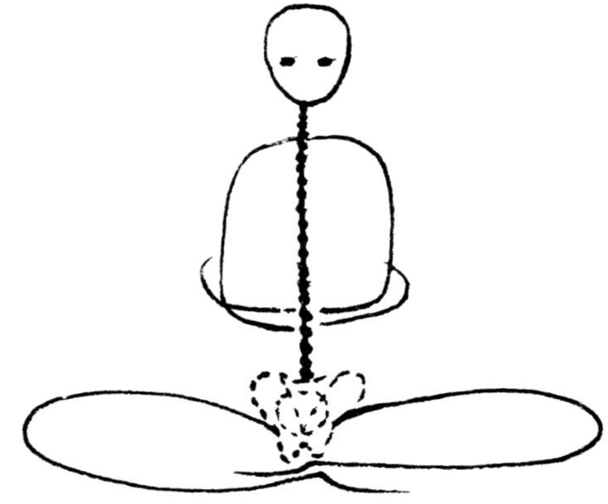

1. Sit in easy position. Arms folded behind back.

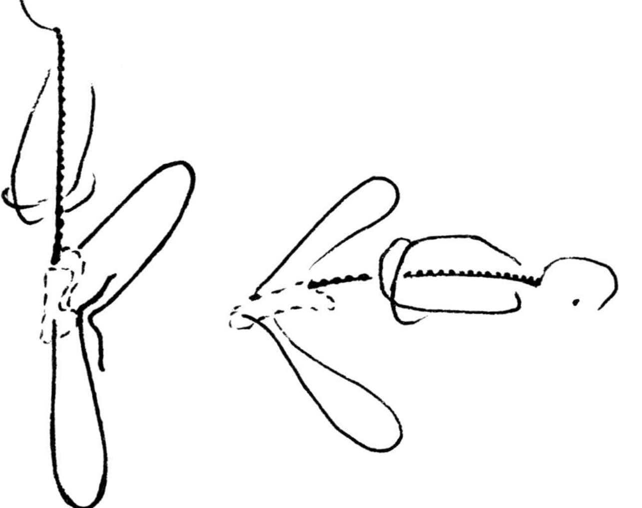

2. Bend forward from the hips, keeping spine straight. Chestbone stretches forward until forehead rests on floor. Keep both buttocks on floor. Then lock up, hollowing spine and stretching chin forward.

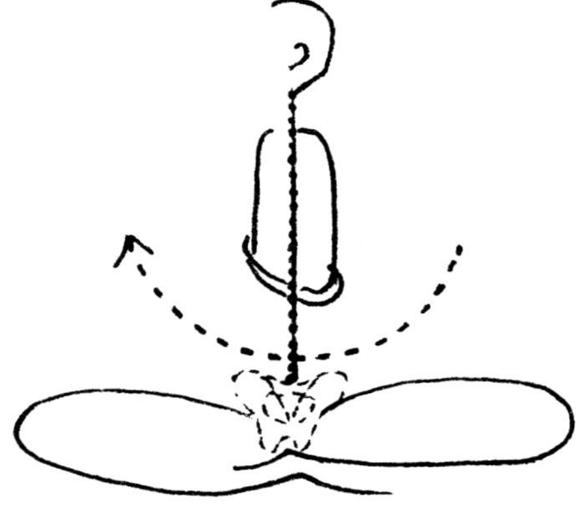

3. Return to easy position. Twist trunk to look over right shoulder. Then bring left shoulder to touch left knee.
   Come up and repeat on other side. Buttocks remain on floor throughout.

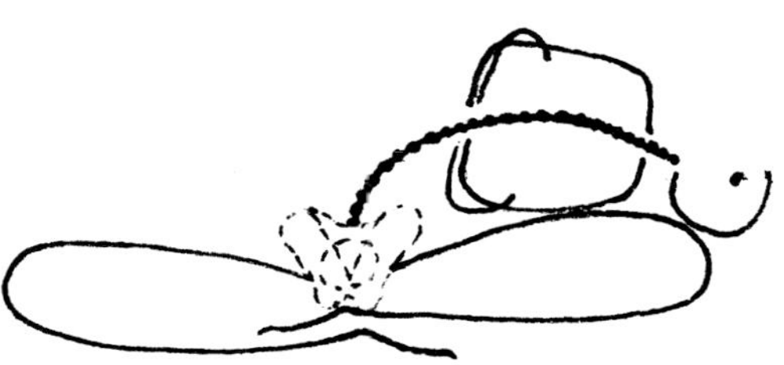

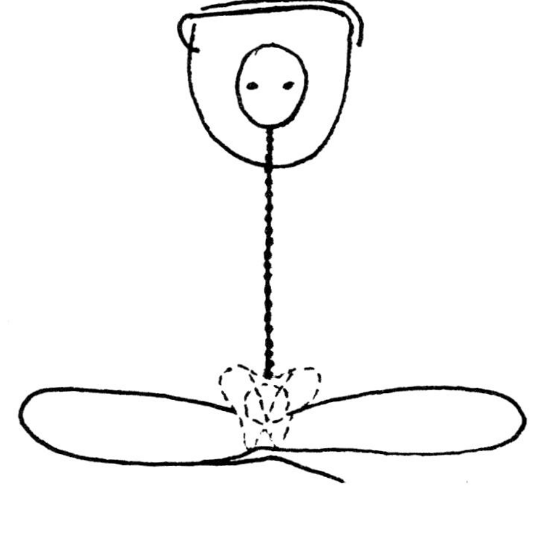

EXERCISE XVI

1. Repeat exercises on p. 58 holding on to elbows above head.

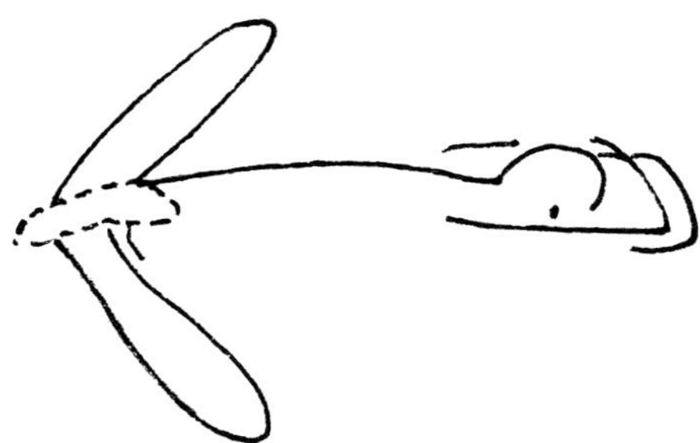

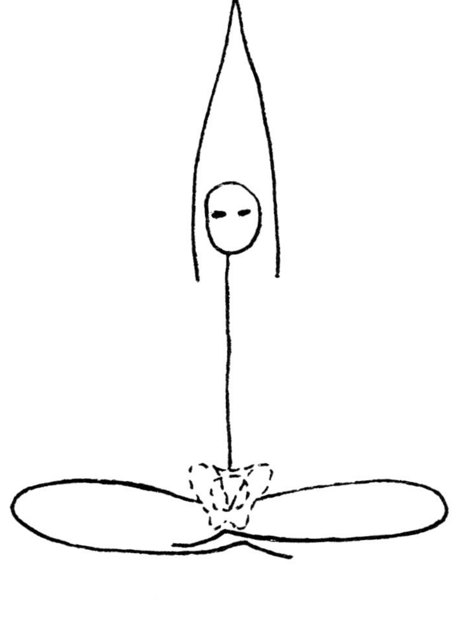

2. Repeat with arms straight above head, palms together.

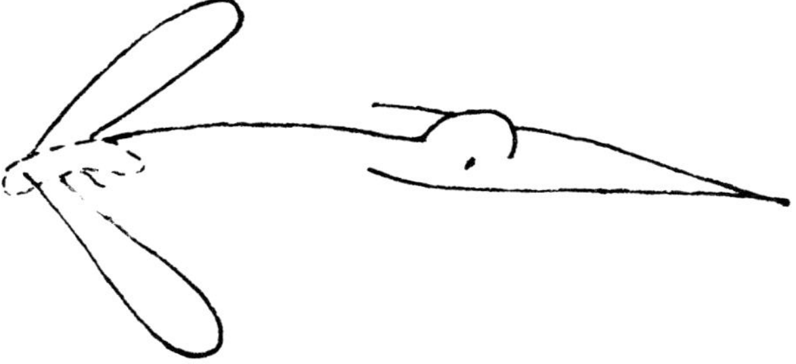

5. Pelvis, Hips and Buttocks

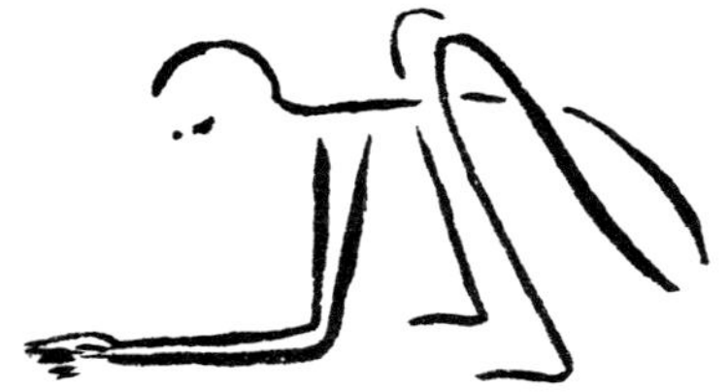

EXERCISE XVII

1. Stand with feet one foot apart, toes pointed forward. Squat down. Keep heels on floor. Spread knees. Bring elbows and hands together. Gently bounce up and down. Elbows and hands should contact the floor. Repeat many times.

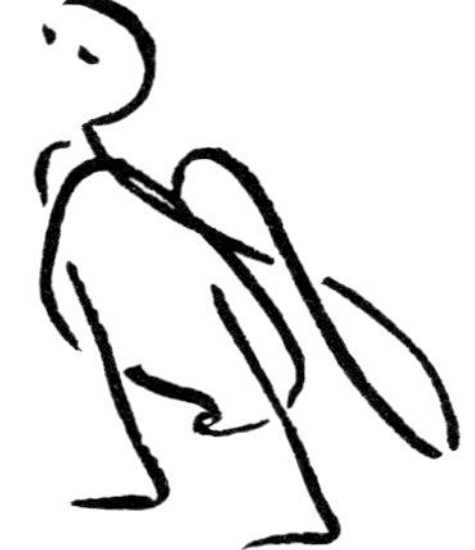

2. Bring upper arms in front of shins and hands round the outside of the ankles. Interlace fingers behind ankles, or hold on to back of heels. Hollow spine. Look up at ceiling.

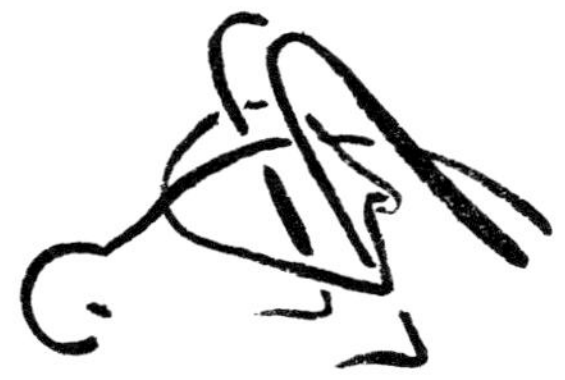

3. Then rounding spine, pull head toward floor. Hold as long as comfortable.

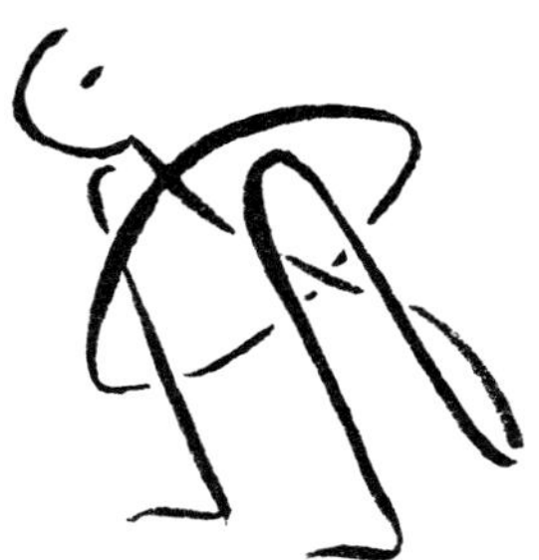

4. Release grip on fingers or foot. Keeping right arm in front of shin, place top of right hand on the back. Move left arm behind back and hold right hand with left hand. Increase grip until you can hold wrist. Straighten spine. Turn trunk so that left side of chest is upward. Look over left shoulder straight behind you. Hold.
   Release grip and repeat this step with other arm.

5. Squat down and maintaining this position, walk through room. Make sure that with each step heel contacts floor. Keep buttocks as close to floor as possible.

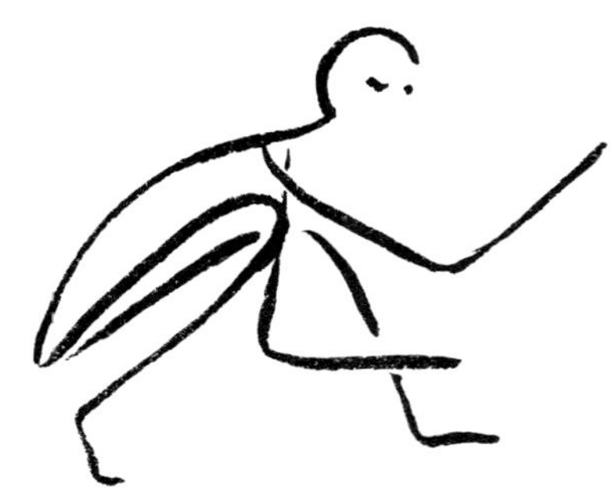

5. Pelvis, Hips and Buttocks

EXERCISE XVIII

1. Stand with feet four to five feet apart, toes pointed forward. Come down squatting on right leg, right foot pointed forward, heel on floor. Left leg is straight, foot flat on floor and pointed forward. Bring elbows and hands together. Bounce elbows toward floor. Right shoulder sinks down inside right knee. Repeat squatting on left leg.

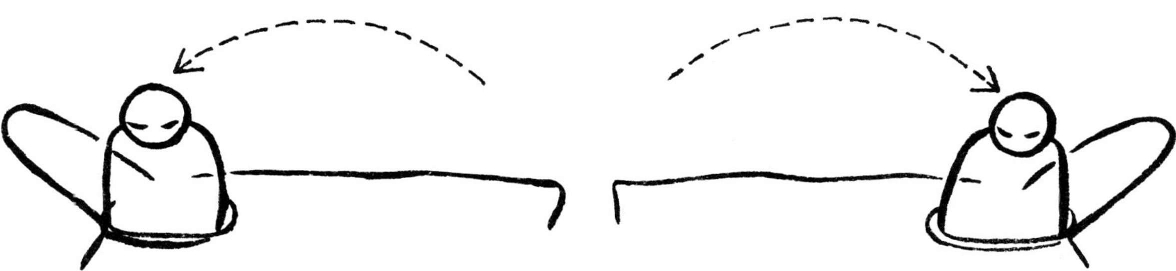

2. Assume above position, but hold on to elbows. Move from right to left and left to right, alternately squatting on right and left feet. Keep bottom as low as possible during movement. Repeat many times.

EXERCISE XIX

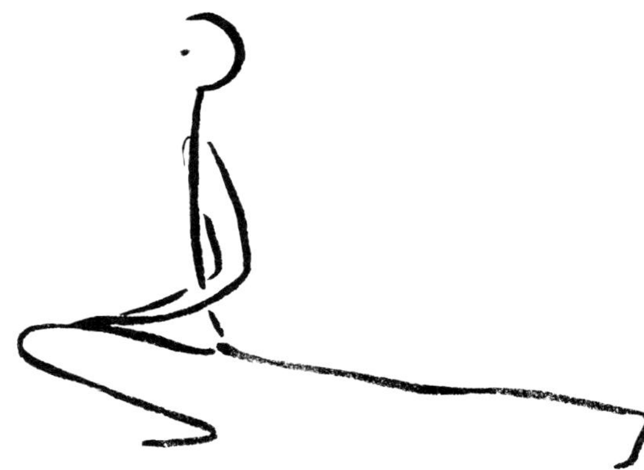

1. Kneel down. Place right foot flat on floor in front of you, toes pointed forward. Stretch left leg backward, keeping it straight. Tuck toes of left foot under. Right buttock sinks down as close as possible to right heel, which remains in contact with floor. Rest both hands on top of right thigh. Straighten spine. Gently bounce up and down. Repeat on other side.

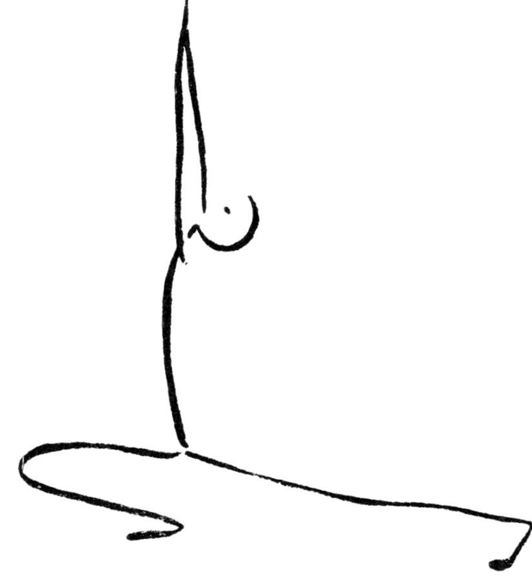

2. In this position, raise both arms above head. Bring palms together; lock thumbs. Keeping arms straight, move them backward, elbows behind ears. Drop head backward and look up at ceiling past thumbs. Balance. Repeat on other side.

EXERCISE XX

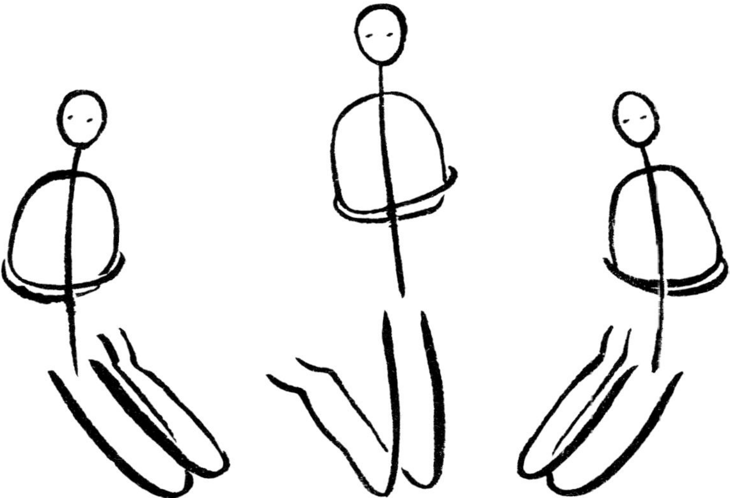

Kneel down, insides of ankles touching, feet on floor. Cross arms behind back. Then sit on floor to the left of your feet. Return to starting position and sit on floor to the right of your feet. Return to starting position. Repeat many times.

EXERCISE XXI

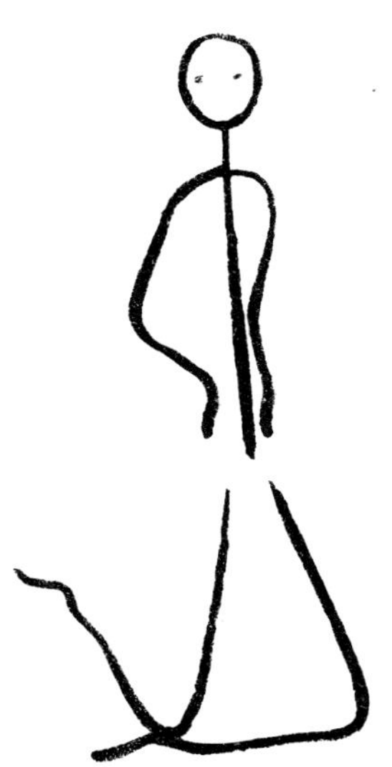

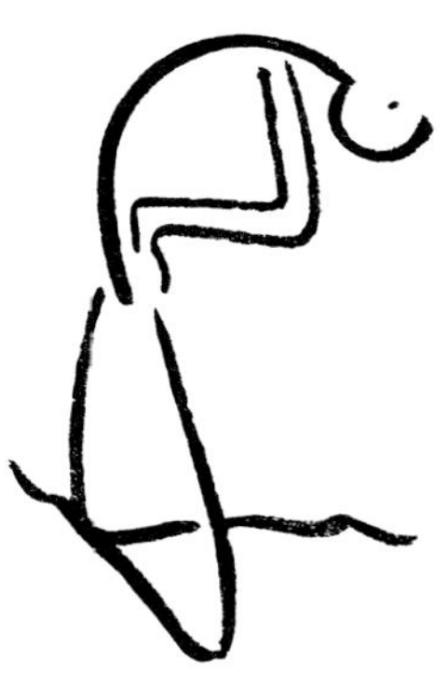

1. Kneel on floor. Place outside of left ankle against right knee so that sole of left foot faces up. Left knee should be on floor in line with right knee. Hands on back of the hips.

2. Push pelvis forward. Arch spine. Bend backward, dropping head to look at wall behind you. Hold. Come up and repeat with other foot in front.

EXERCISE XXII

1. Sit on floor with right leg straight and as far to the right as possible. Bend left knee so that left foot curls around left buttock, top of foot on floor, sole facing upward. Place both hands on floor in front of you. Move trunk forward; chestbone moves toward floor. Keep both buttocks on floor.

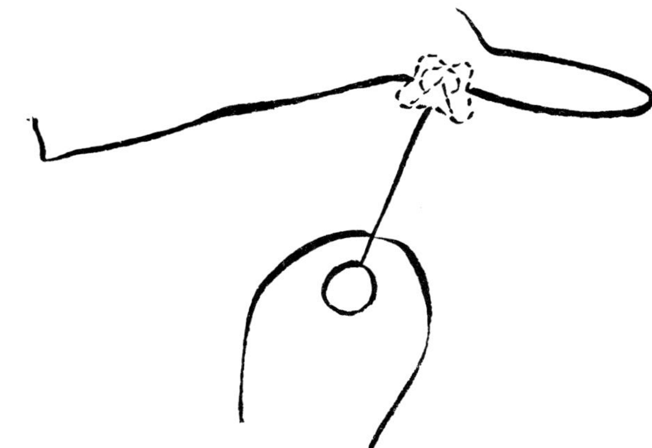

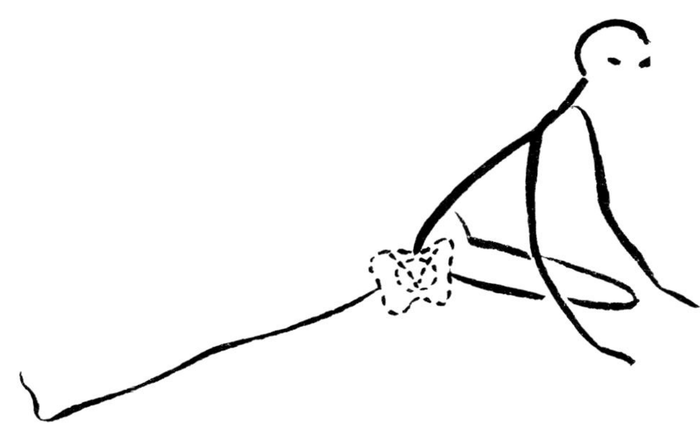

2. Come up to sitting position. Move chestbone toward left knee. Keep both buttocks on floor. Repeat both steps with other leg bent.

EXERCISE XXIII

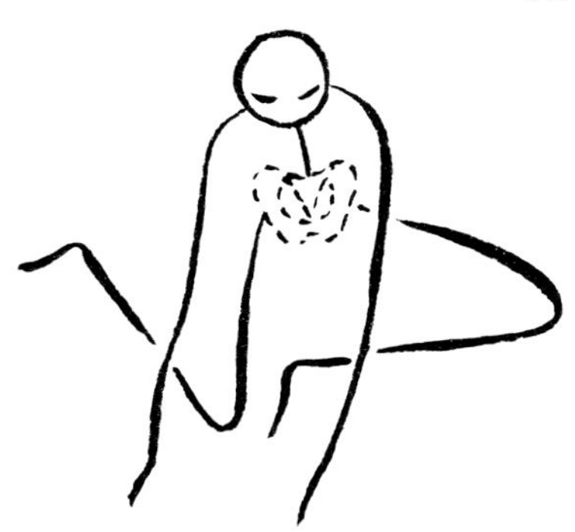

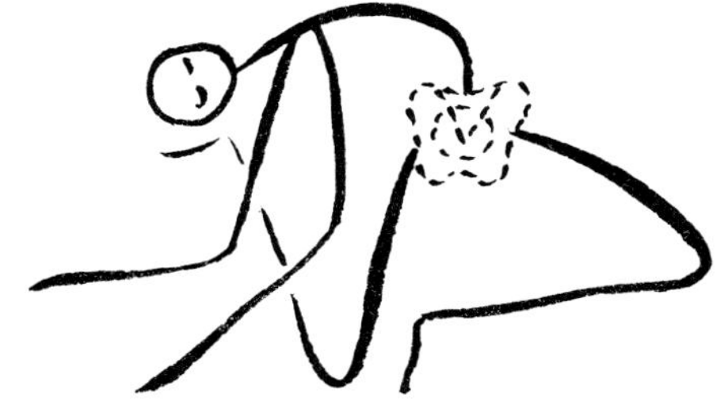

1. Sit on floor. Bend knees and drop them both to floor towards the left. Sole of left foot touches inside of right thigh. Bring chestbone forward over right thigh and knee.

2. Return to sitting position. Then move sideways and twist so that right elbow moves toward floor. Keep both buttocks on floor.
Repeat both steps on other side.

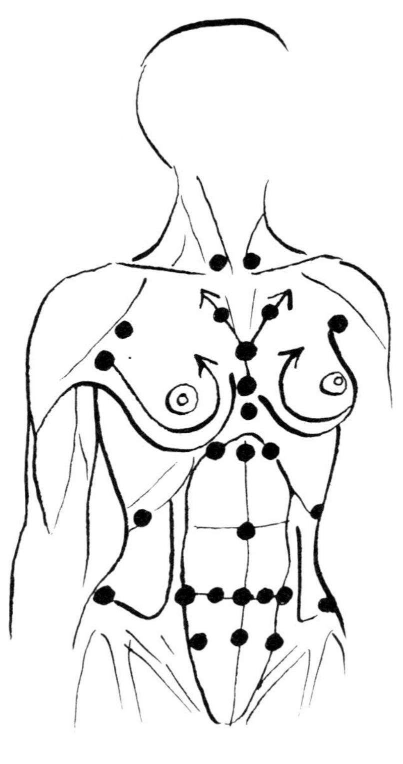

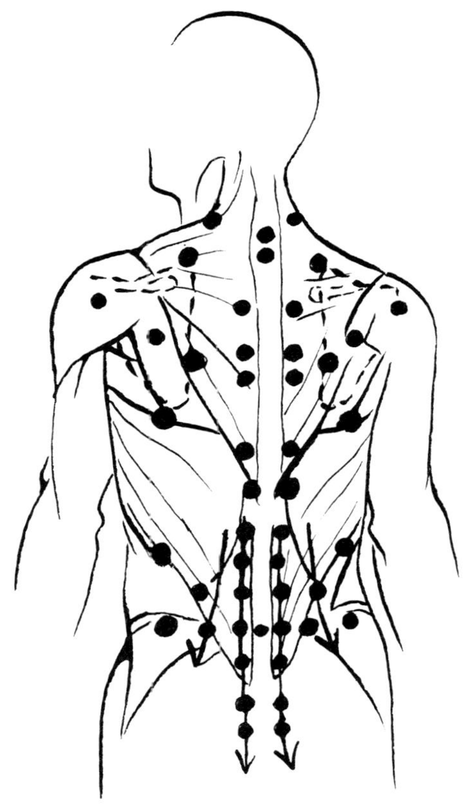

6. BACK, SPINE AND ABDOMEN

This chapter focuses on the back and spine and posture, though it also contains numerous exercises for the abdomen and chest. If you consider the whole area as the trunk, you will understand better the interconnectedness of spine and back with chest and abdomen in front, pelvis and hips below, shoulders and neck above. The segments of the living body cannot be arbitrarily dissociated from each other.

The spine consists of 24 true vertebrae, separated by discs or pads of cartilaginous fibre allowing some movement between them. There are seven cervical, twelve thoracic, and five lumbar vertebrae. The last nine vertebrae are called false vertebrae, since they are so closely fused together as to make movement between them virtually impossible. There are twelve ribs, though only the first seven are joined to the chestbone (see p. 48) as well as to the thoracic vertebrae. The 24 vertebrae are capable of backward, forward, and sideways, as well as twisting, movement. The exercise you did on p. 12, plus those on pp. 66 and 72, give you a sense of your spine and its vertebral components.

A supple spine is essential for good health. Standing erect does not mean standing straight as a board, but standing so that the spine assumes its natural position without effort or tension. No muscles are needed to push or pull the spine if it is in the proper position. You will be able to feel when the spine is properly situated in relation to the head and shoulders above, the pelvis and legs below, and the muscles and organs inside, feeling neither strain nor cramp. As the spine is the protector and container of the bulk of the central nervous system, an uninterrupted flow of energy must be available. When people speak of a pinched nerve in the back, they mean that it is pinched between two vertebrae.

The forward bend exercises stretch the back muscles, while the backward bend stretches the abdominal and pelvic muscles as well as strengthening the back muscles. The abdominal muscles must be strong, but not tight, in order to allow for deep and unrestricted breathing. As explained in the introduction to Chapter 4, you may feel strain or fatigue when beginning. Respond with massage and gentle flexing of the affected area. Then continue the exercise comfortably over a period of time, remembering that true strength comes from true relaxation. The twist exercises give the whole trunk area an excellent workout, combining strength, stretching, and balance.

THE SPINE SEEN FROM THE LEFT SIDE

ATLAS
AXIS

NECK

7TH CERVICAL
1ST THORACIC

UPPER AND MIDDLE
PART OF BACK

12TH THORACIC
1ST LUMBAR

LOWER BACK

5TH LUMBAR

SACRUM

TAILBONE

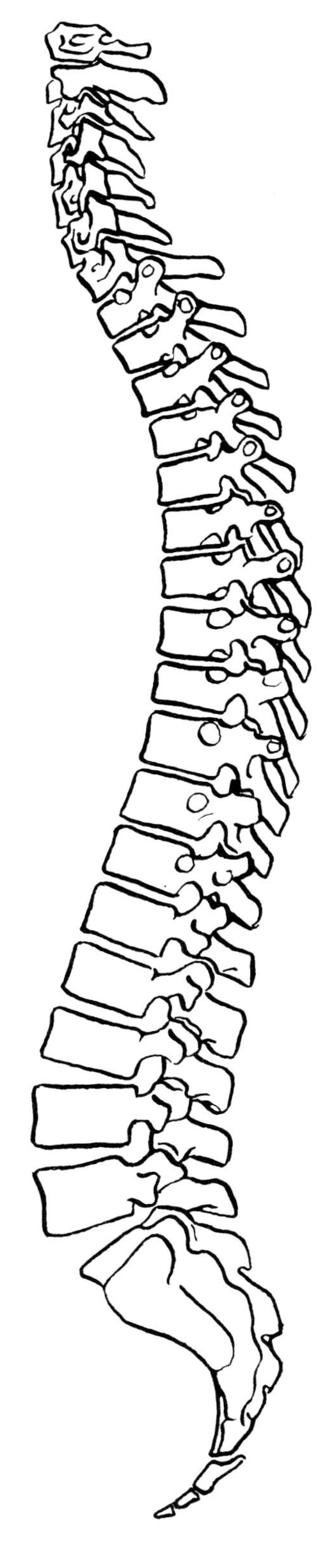

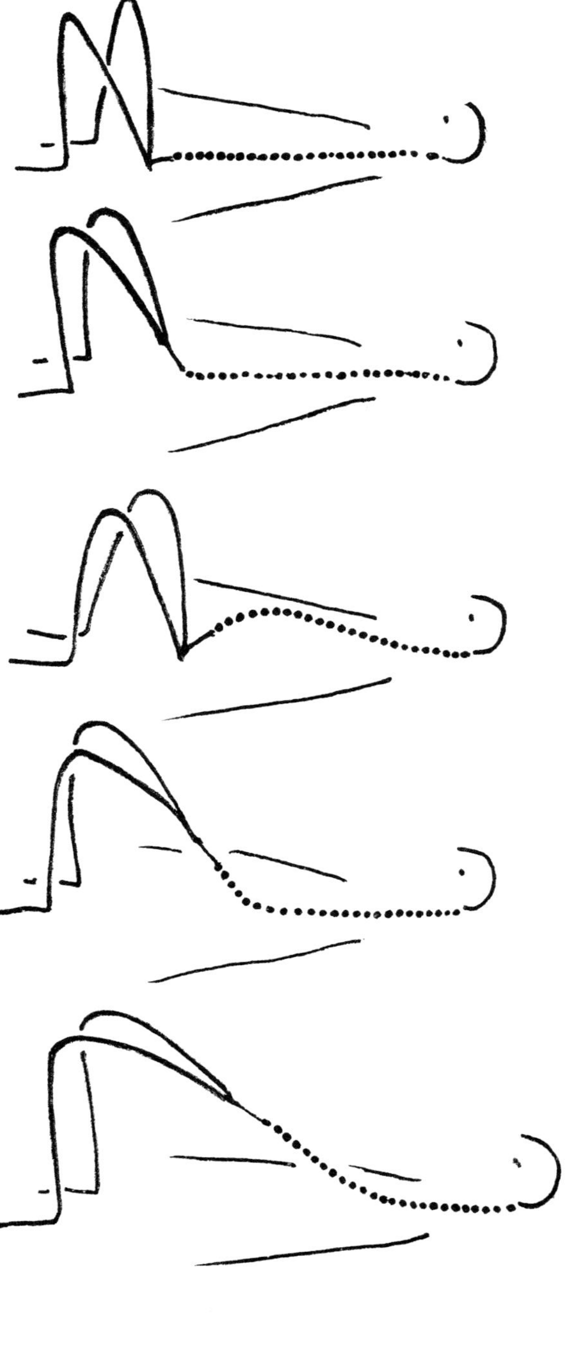

EXERCISE I

1. Lie down on floor and feel how spine contacts floor. Place feet about one foot away from buttocks, feet one foot apart, heels under knees.

2. Lift tailbone (4 fused vertebrae) and sacrum (5 fused vertebrae) off floor. Put them back down as in picture 1.

3. Now arch spine so lower and middle back come off floor. Tailbone remains in contact with floor. Put spine back down on floor, as in picture 1.

4. Lift tailbone, sacrum, and first vertebra in lower back off floor. Put spine back down (picture 1), arch spine (picture 3), and return spine to floor again (picture 1).

5. Repeat movements each time lifting one more vertebra off floor. This picture shows 12 vertebrae off floor. End up supporting body on feet and neck vertebrae. Arms relaxed. Rest when tired.
   Then put spine back down, reversing movements vertebra by vertebra.

6. Now assume position of supporting body on feet and neck vertebrae. Move knees and head from right to left repeating many times until movement is flowing. Keep pushing pelvis upward. Relax.
   Now, move knees to right and head to left; then head to right and knees to left. Push pelvis upward. Coordinate movement. Relax and lie down flat. Feel how back contacts floor.

EXERCISE II

1. Lie on floor, arms next to body. Move awareness to your back. Feel how it contacts floor. Place feet a comfortable distance away from buttocks, one foot apart. Relax legs. Cross left leg over right.

2. Move right knee to the left toward floor. Right shoulder remains on floor. Move knee back up. Repeat 25 times with easy and relaxed movement. Feel how back contacts floor. Repeat 25 times with other leg crossed.

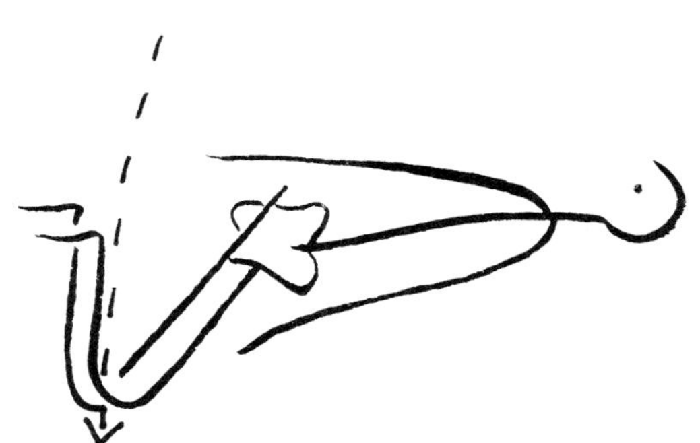

3. Begin as in picture 2, right knee on or close to floor. Then interlock fingers behind base of skull.

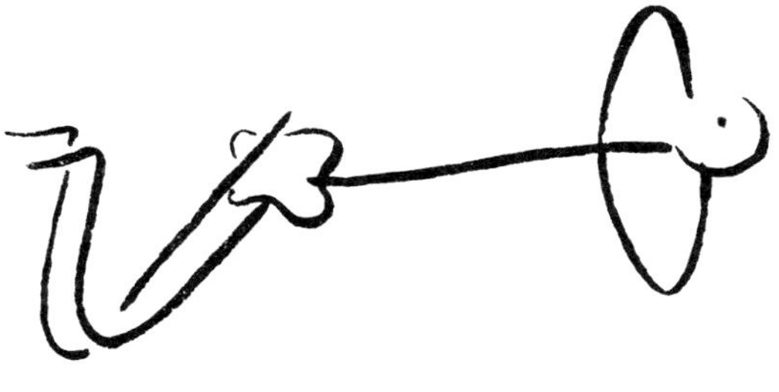

4. Lift shoulders, so that upper part of back and head are off floor. Elbows point forward. Look over right hip. Keeping knees in position, put back elbows, shoulders, and head down on floor. Repeat 25 times. Repeat with other leg.

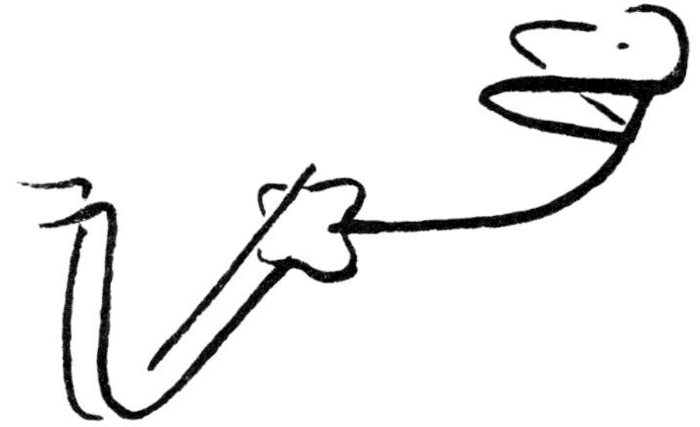

EXERCISE III

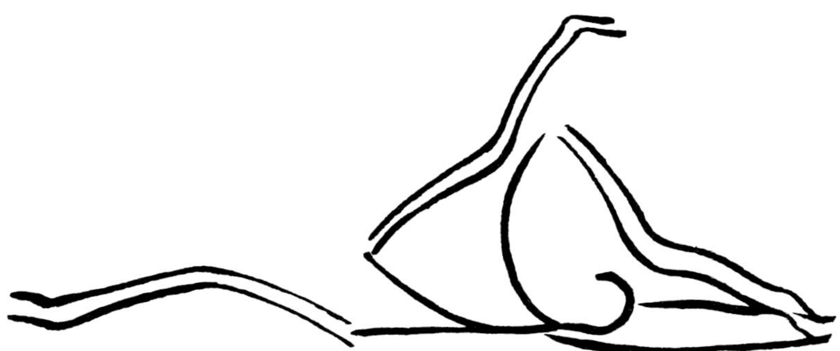

Lie down on your back, legs together, arms over head on floor. Swing both legs over head. Toes touch floor for a moment and spine comes off floor. Roll spine in reverse movement back on floor and lie down again for a moment. Then swing legs over head again.
Repeat this rising and falling movement many times.

EXERCISE IV

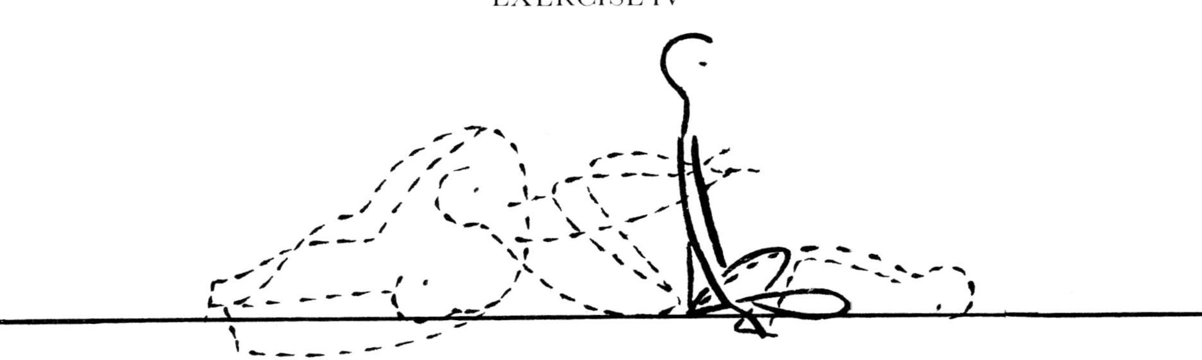

Sit cross-legged on floor. Right hand takes left foot. Left hand takes right foot. Roll backward, keeping spine round and soft. Feet move over head to touch floor for a moment and then come back over head, movement flowing so as to return to sitting position, but let momentum continue so that forehead moves forward and touches the floor, while keeping buttocks on floor. Then come up and begin backward roll again.
Repeat many times with right leg in front, then change to left leg in front. Movement should be flowing and easy.

EXERCISE V

1. Lie down on stomach, left cheek on floor, arms over head on floor.

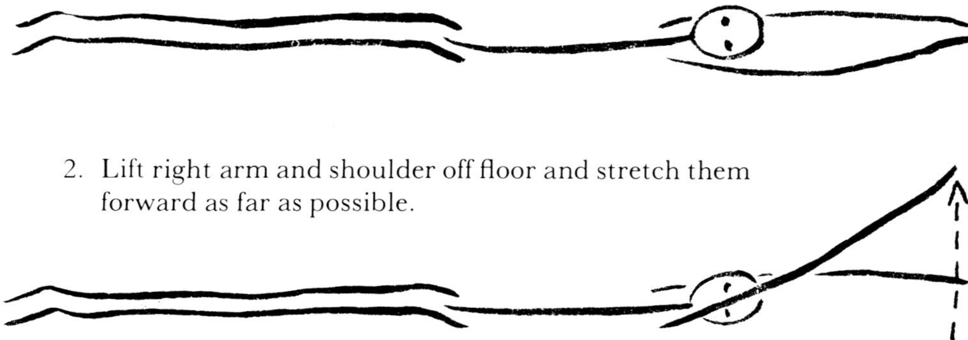

2. Lift right arm and shoulder off floor and stretch them forward as far as possible.

3. Put right arm back down while lifting left leg off floor. Stretch leg backward. When arm goes down, leg comes up; when leg goes down, arm comes up. Repeat this many times and on other side.

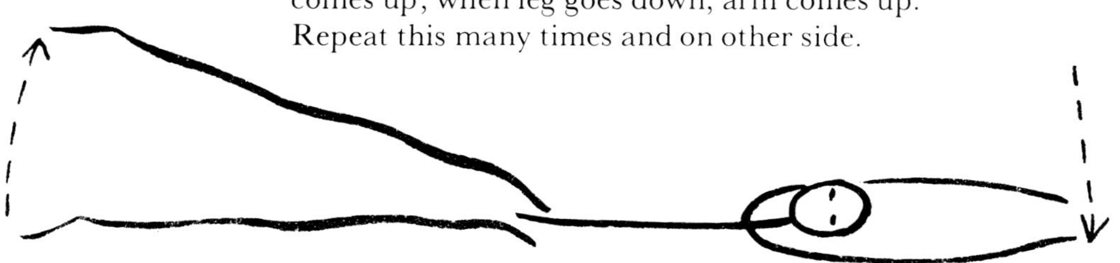

4. Then lift right shoulder and arm, head, and left leg off floor. Look up at ceiling. Keep left arm and right leg relaxed. Repeat several times. Rest right cheek on floor and repeat on other side.

EXERCISE VI

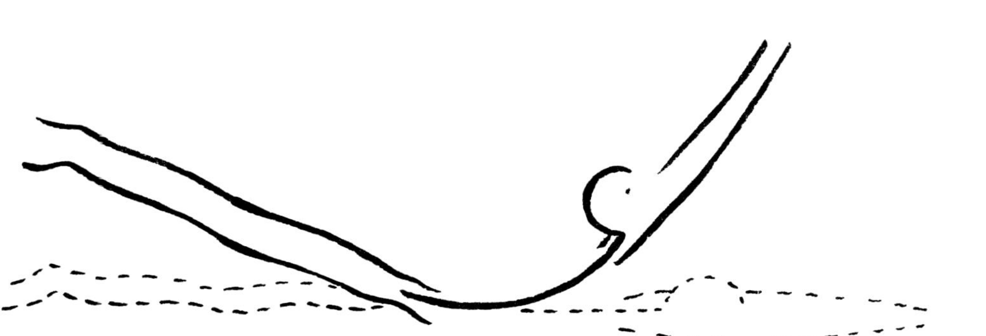

Lie down facing floor, arms stretched above head on floor. Stretch arms and legs upward, so that only abdomen and hipbones contact floor. Arch spine. Keep legs and arms straight. Hold as long as comfortable. Then relax. Repeat three times.

EXERCISE VII:
MONKEY WALK

1. Walk on all fours like a monkey, fast and slow. Observe how arms and legs coordinate. Continue for at least five minutes.

EXERCISE VIII: CAT WALK

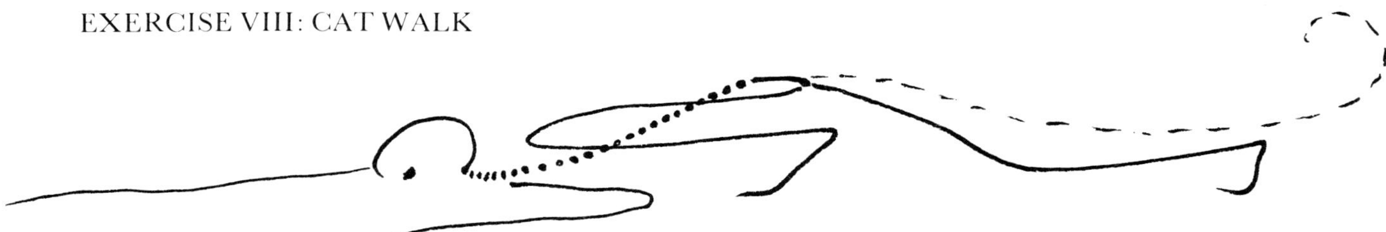

Walk on all fours, sinking through elbows and knees, chest close to floor. Observe coordination of hands and feet.

EXERCISE IX: LIZARD WALK

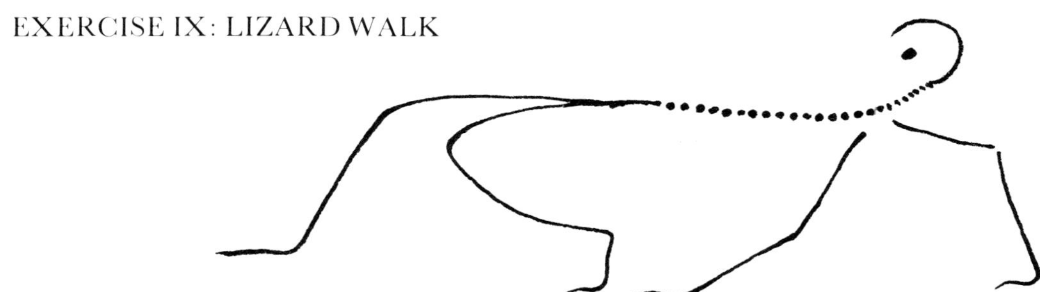

Sit on floor, legs straight. Place hands behind buttocks on floor. Lift pelvis off floor. Walk ten steps forward and ten steps backward, pushing pelvis upward.

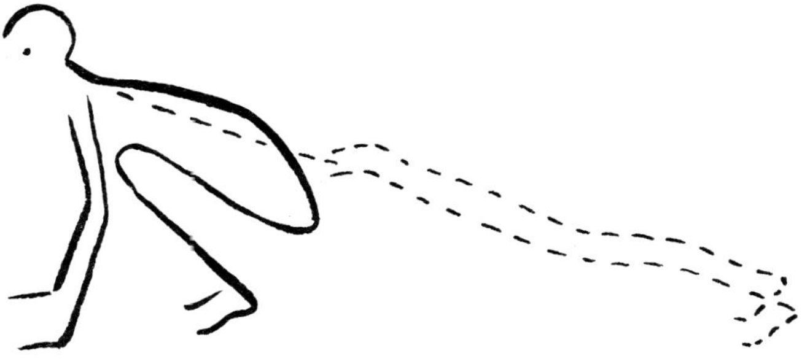

EXERCISE X

Squat down on toes. Hands on floor in line with shoulders. Jump backward, straightening legs and landing lightly on toes. Legs and back form one straight line. Arms at right angle to floor. Jump forward and backward many times.

EXERCISE XI

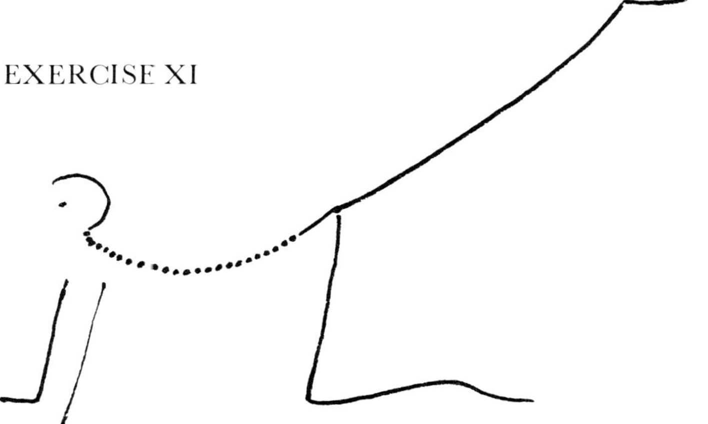

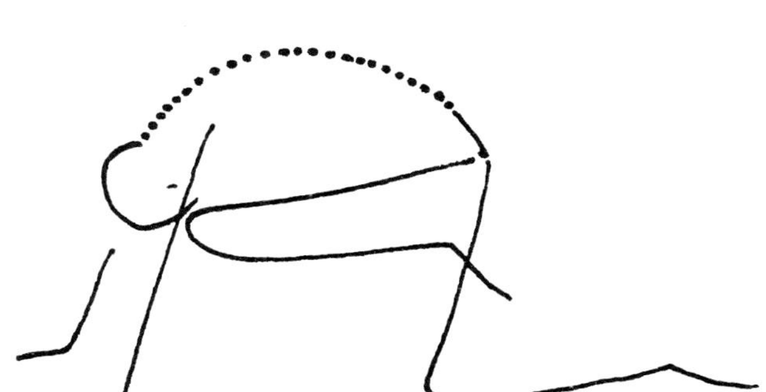

1. Knee. on all fours. Stretch right leg backward and upward. Hollow spine. Look up.

2. Return through kneeling position with right leg, drawing right knee toward forehead, chin against chestbone. Then swing leg backward and upward again.
   Repeat several times with each leg.

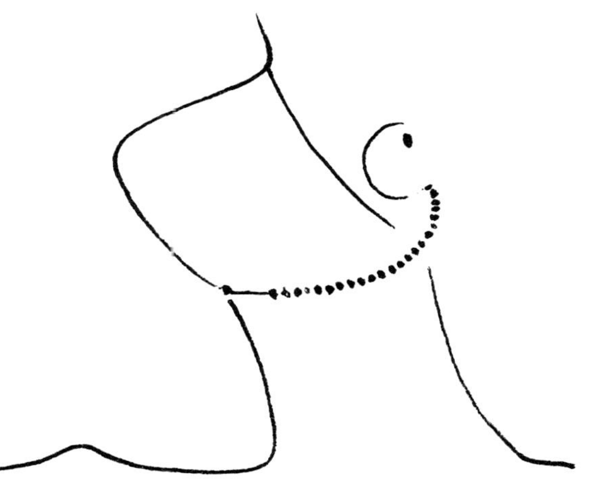

EXERCISE XII

Return to kneeling position, hands in line with shoulders, knees five inches apart. Take right ankle in left hand, raising foot away from buttocks. Hollow back. Look forward and upward. Hold as long as comfortable.
Repeat with other leg.

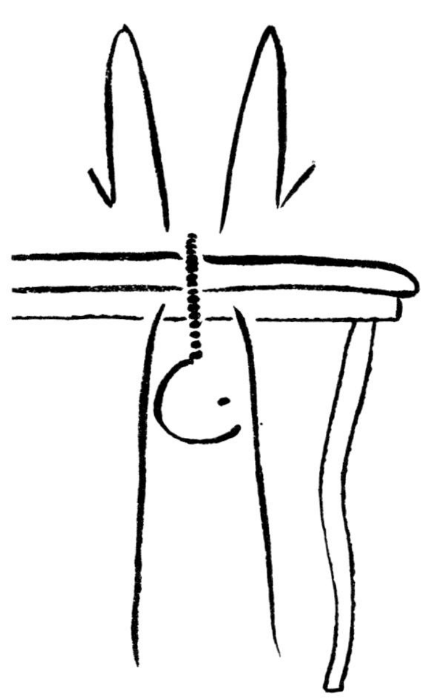

EXERCISE XIII

1. Lie down on a firm table, knees bent. Hang head backward over edge of table. Relax neck. Turn head from right to left many times.

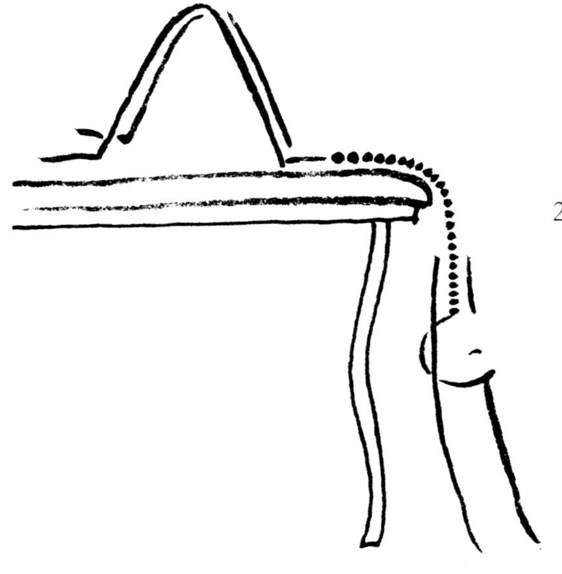

2. Slowly slide back over edge of table, feeling vertebra by vertebra. Let arms hang. Relax back.

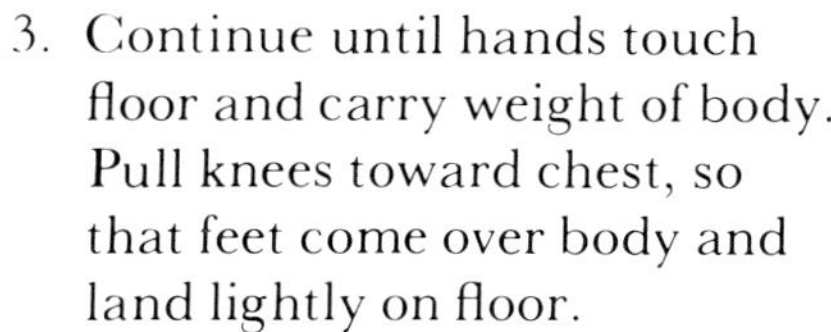

3. Continue until hands touch floor and carry weight of body. Pull knees toward chest, so that feet come over body and land lightly on floor.

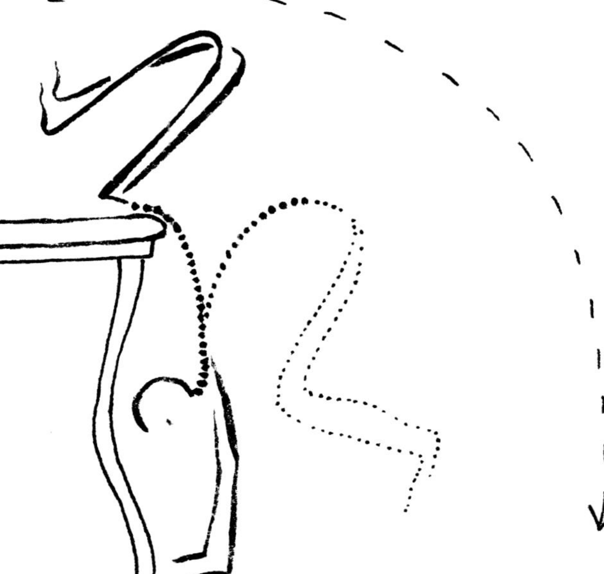

EXERCISE XIV: THE CRAB

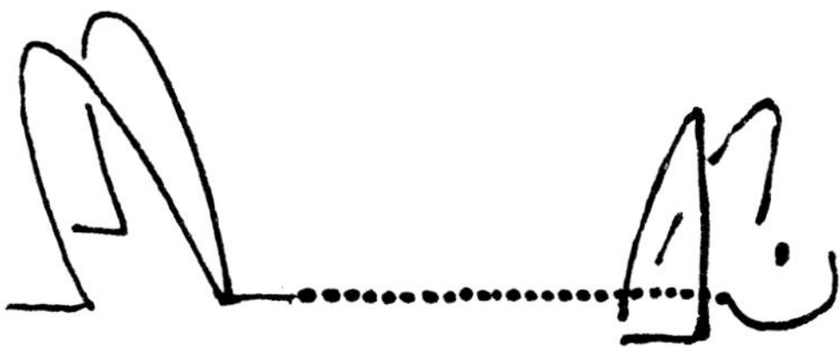

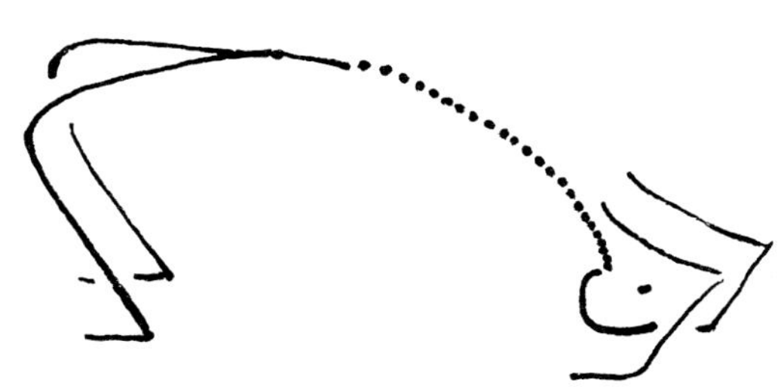

1. Lie down on back. Place feet flat on floor one foot apart, as close to buttocks as possible. Hands on floor under shoulders, palms down, fingers pointing toward feet.

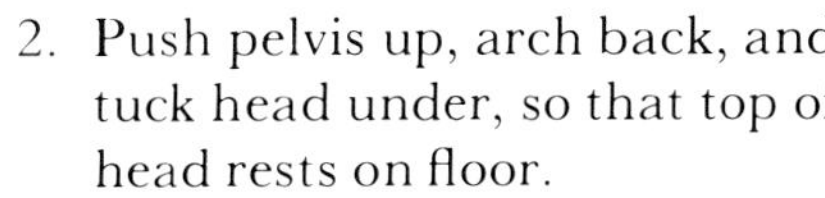

2. Push pelvis up, arch back, and tuck head under, so that top of head rests on floor.

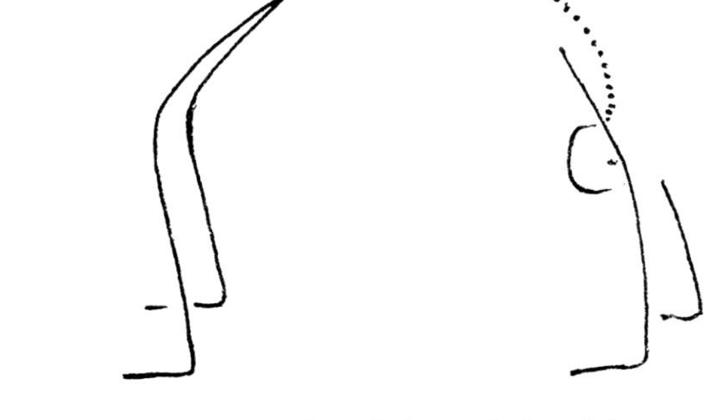

3. Now straighten arms, push pelvis and shoulders upward, so that head comes off floor. (This position can be reached directly from picture 1 by simply straightening arms, arching spine, and pushing pelvis upward.) Hold as long as comfortable.
   When you find this easy, try walking forward and backward, to left and right in this position. When you can do this, try the following variation.

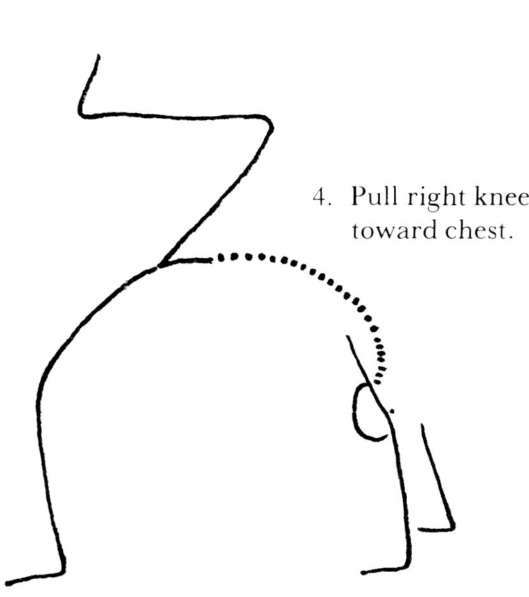

4. Pull right knee toward chest.

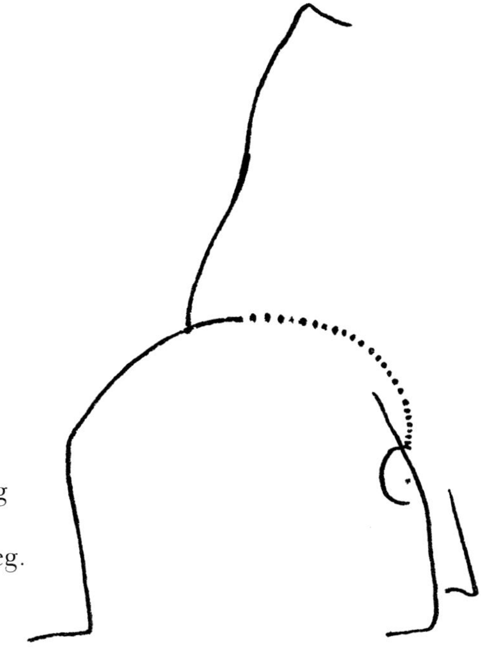

5. Stretch leg upward, heel toward ceiling. Bend knee and bring foot back to floor. Repeat with other leg.

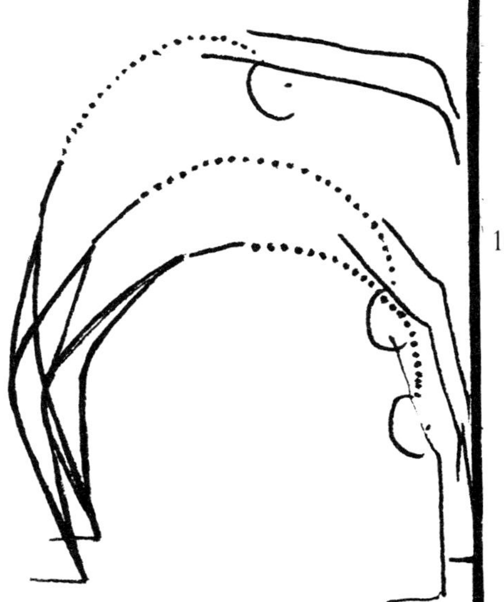

EXERCISE XV: THE BACKWARD BEND

This is not an exercise for beginners.

1. With your back to a wall at a distance of two to three feet, stretch arms over head. Lean backward, placing palms against wall, fingers pointing downward. Walk down wall with hands until hands rest on floor. Now try to walk back up. Repeat several times.

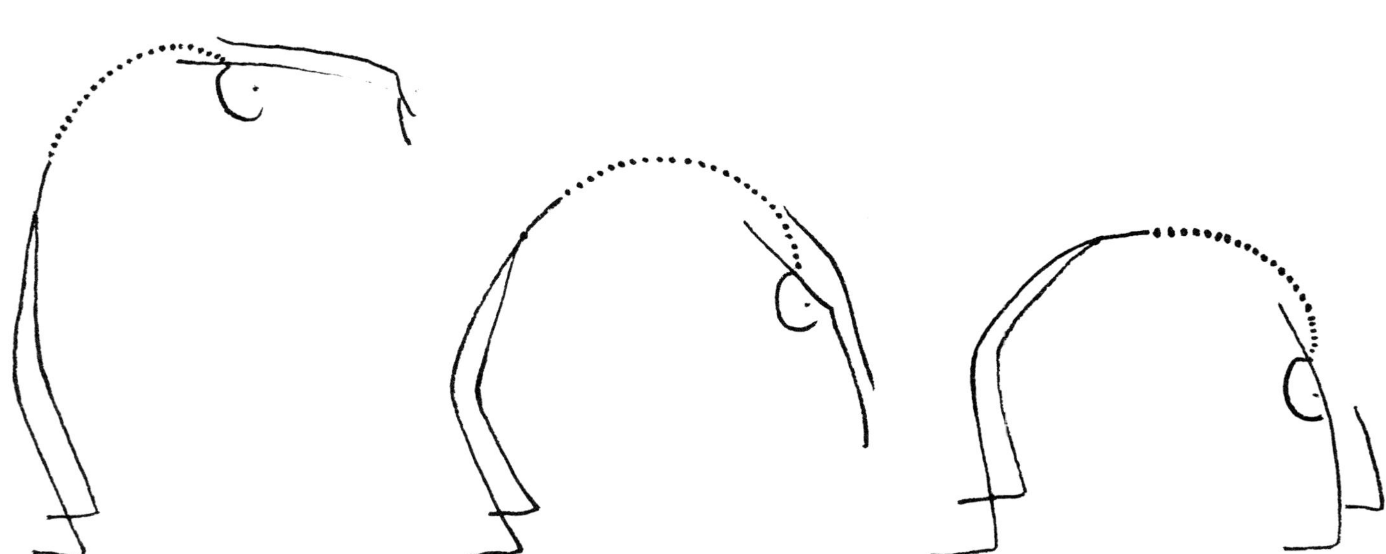

2. Now try without the wall. Stand with feet one foot apart. Stretch arms over head and lean backward. Slowly, without losing control, moving into backward bend. Try to return to standing position.

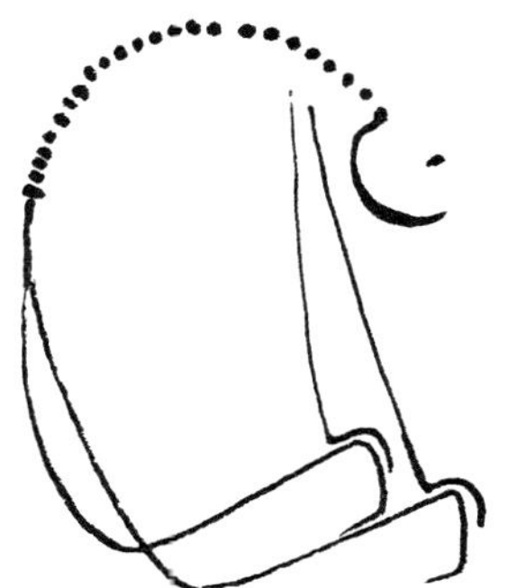

EXERCISE XVI

1. Kneel, knees five inches apart. Tuck toes under. Bend upper spine backward and hold on to both heels, keeping arms straight. Push pelvis forward. Thighs should be at right angle to floor.

2. Repeat exercise with tops of feet on floor. Rest palms of hands on soles of feet.

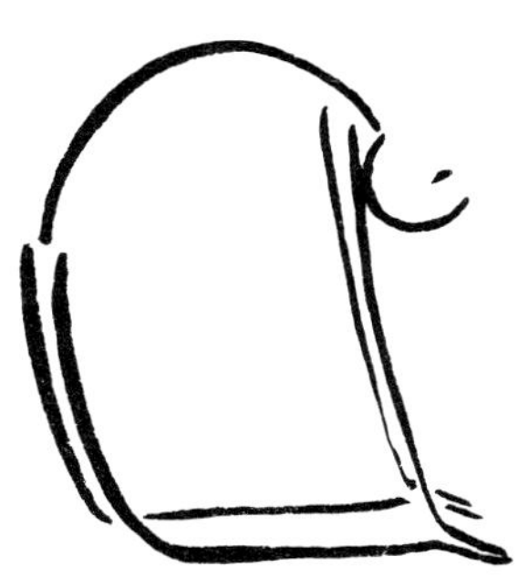

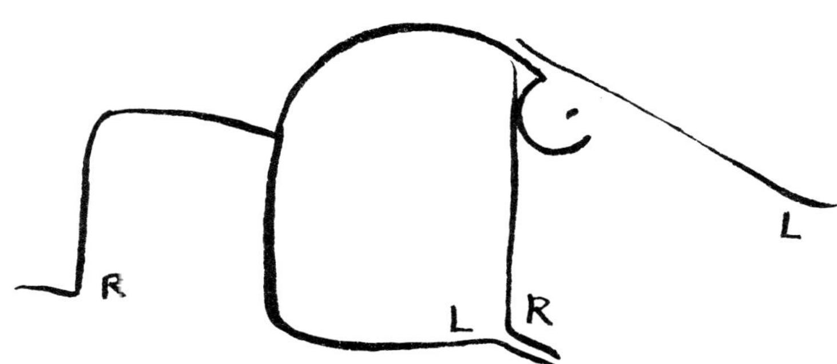

EXERCISE XVII

Kneel on floor. Place right foot flat on floor in front of you. Lean backward and place right hand on back of left ankle or on sole of foot. Stretch left arm backward. Drop head backward. Push pelvis forward. Relax and hold.
Repeat on other side.

EXERCISE XVIII

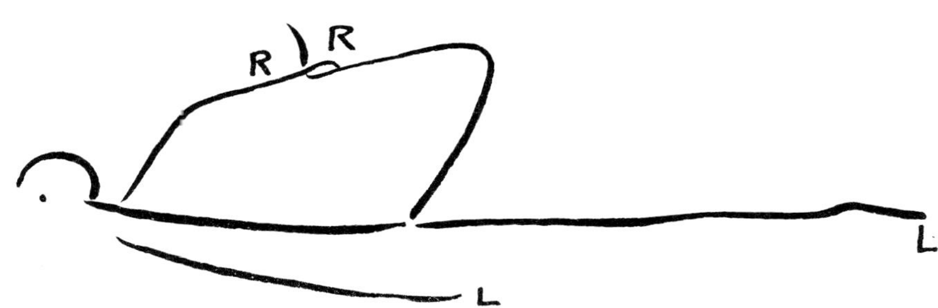

1. Lie down facing floor, arms at your side. Take right ankle in right hand. Move right foot upward while raising thigh off floor. Relax neck and left side of body. Repeat with other leg.

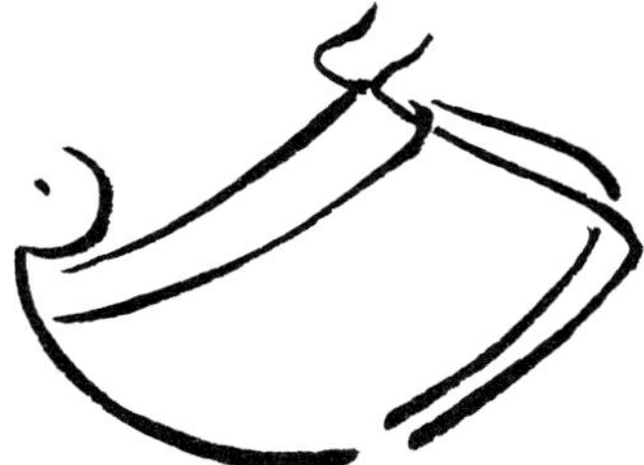

2. Now hold both ankles and stretch legs upward. Body rests on abdomen; chest and thighs are off floor. Arch spine. Look up. Rock forward and backward, massaging intestines and organs of the belly. Coordinate breathing with movements.

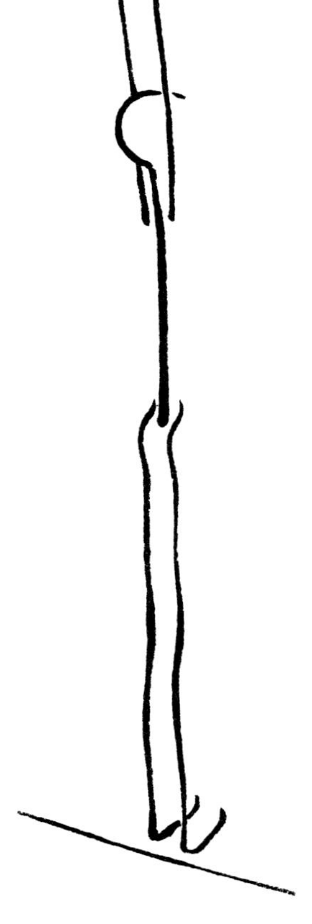

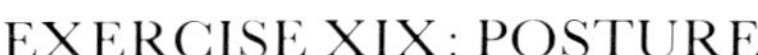

EXERCISE XIX: POSTURE

1. Use a ledge in your home, or place a bar high enough so that you can just grip it. Hang from it. Try to touch floor with one heel, then the other, then both. The spine will stretch. Repeat daily for several minutes.

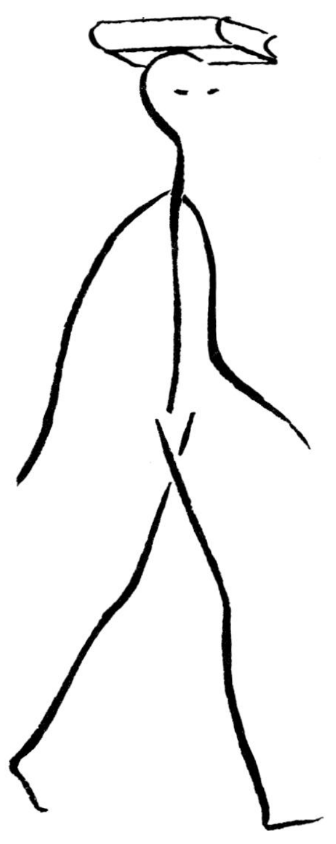

2. Walk around room with a book on your head. While walking, make a conscious effort to stretch your spine.

3. Stand with back against a wall, feet about four inches apart, toes forward. Insteps of feet off floor. The weight of the body is distributed over the whole of the foot. The big toe should not touch the second toe. Knees should be bent slightly and relaxed. Tuck tailbone forward. Straighten spine and bring whole of spine in contact with wall, lower back, middle part of back, upper part of back, and neck if possible. Shoulders move backward and downward, base of skull moves upward. Relax arms.
Move away from wall and walk around room. Go back to wall. Check your posture.

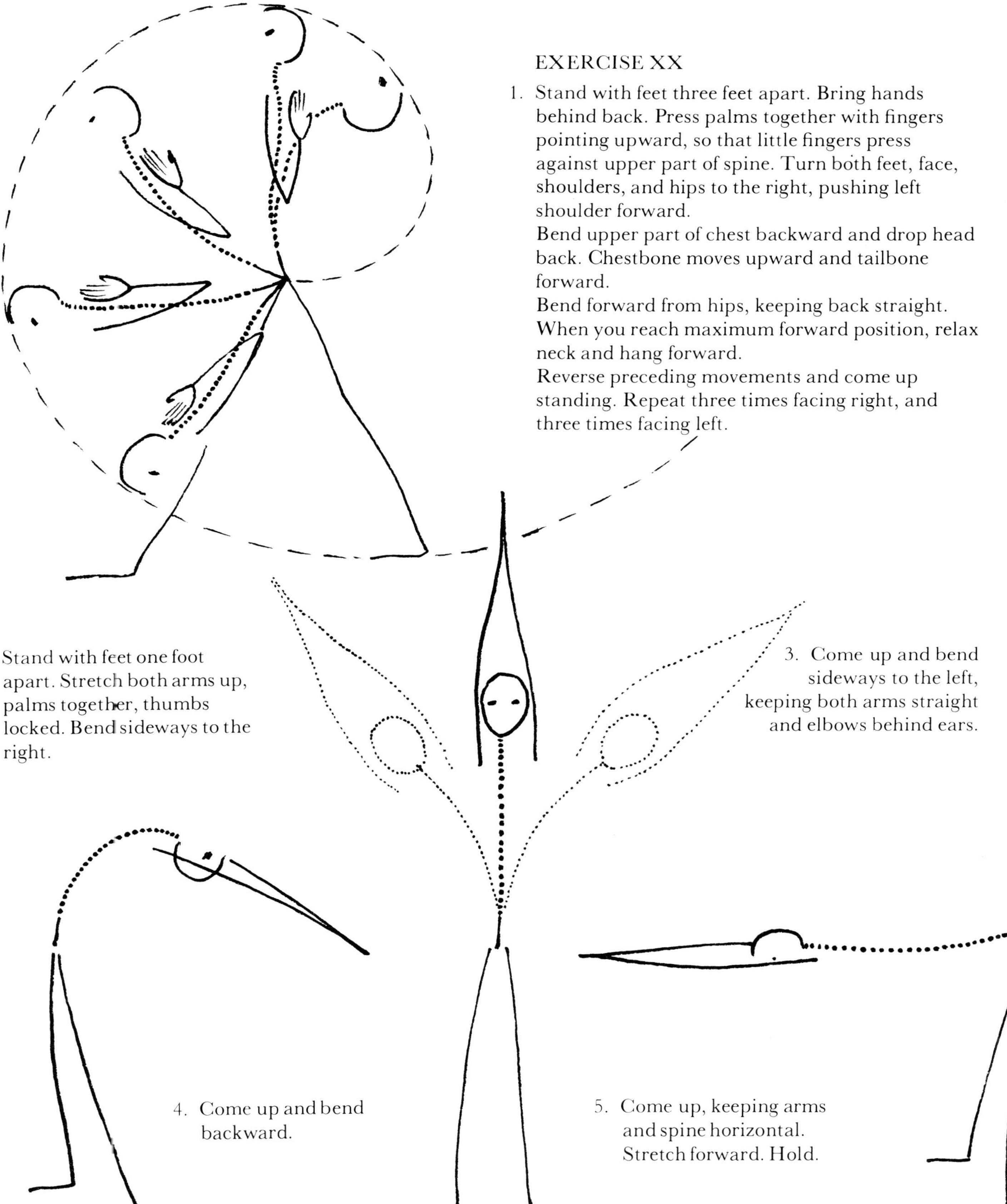

EXERCISE XX

1. Stand with feet three feet apart. Bring hands behind back. Press palms together with fingers pointing upward, so that little fingers press against upper part of spine. Turn both feet, face, shoulders, and hips to the right, pushing left shoulder forward.
   Bend upper part of chest backward and drop head back. Chestbone moves upward and tailbone forward.
   Bend forward from hips, keeping back straight. When you reach maximum forward position, relax neck and hang forward.
   Reverse preceding movements and come up standing. Repeat three times facing right, and three times facing left.

2. Stand with feet one foot apart. Stretch both arms up, palms together, thumbs locked. Bend sideways to the right.

3. Come up and bend sideways to the left, keeping both arms straight and elbows behind ears.

4. Come up and bend backward.

5. Come up, keeping arms and spine horizontal. Stretch forward. Hold.

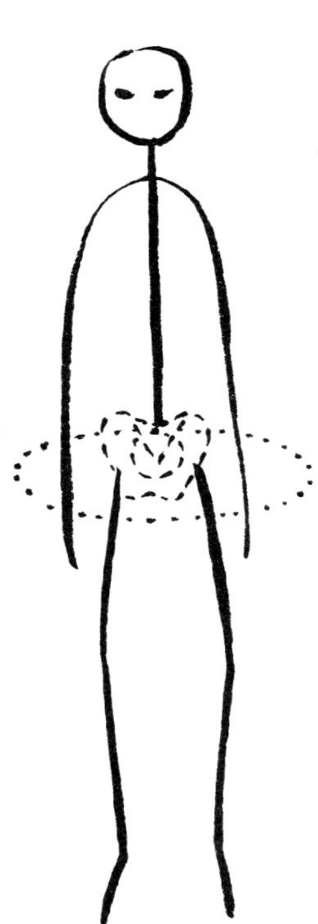

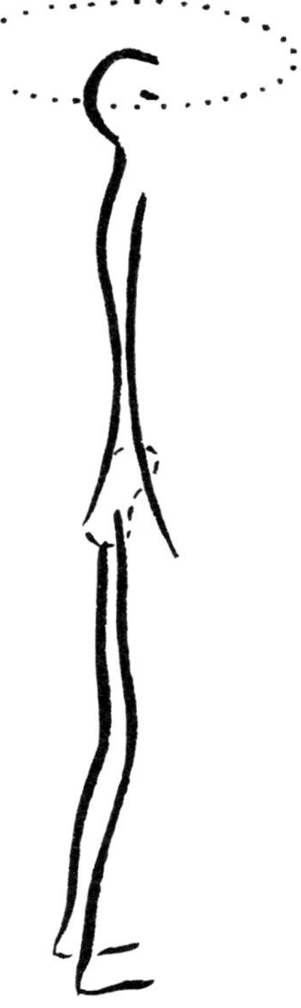

EXERCISE XXI: THE HOUR-GLASS

1. Stand with feet one foot apart, back relaxed. Concentrate on top of head and tailbone. Move pelvis around as if describing a circle on floor with tailbone. Turn clockwise and anti-clockwise. Continue until movement is flowing and easy.
2. Then drop head forward and relax neck. Turn head around as if describing a circle on ceiling with top of head.
3. More tailbone and pelvis forward. Drop head forward as well. Move tailbone and top of head in same circular motion, clockwise and anti-clockwise, slow and fast.

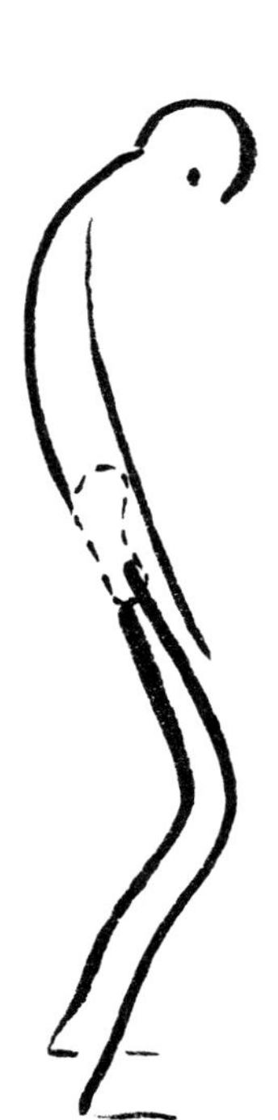

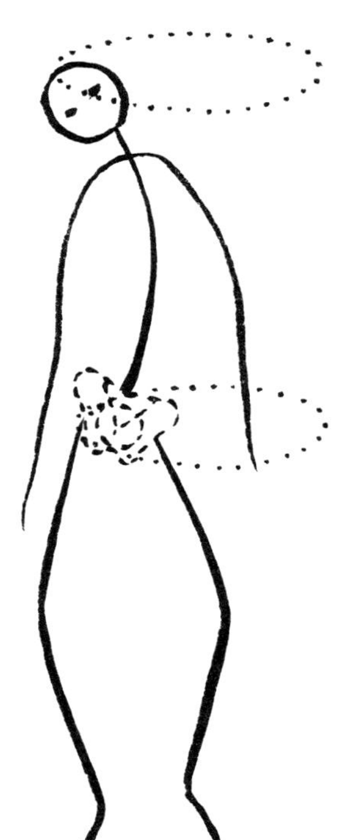

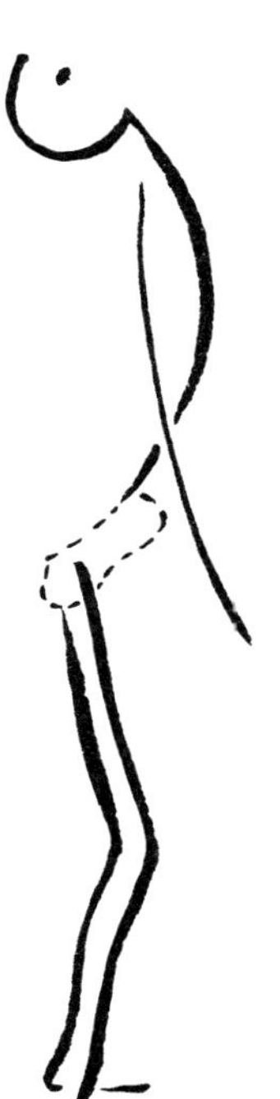

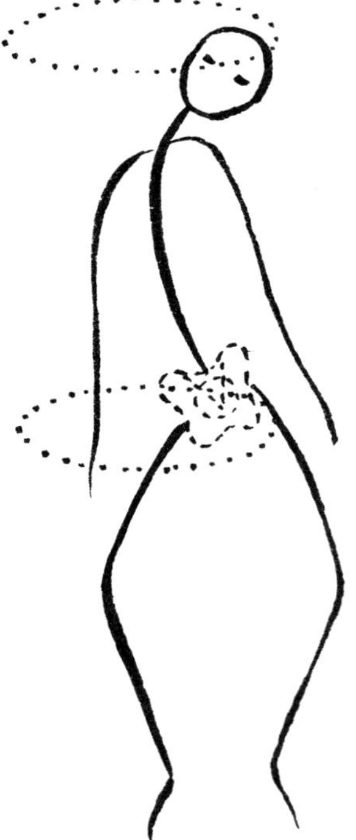

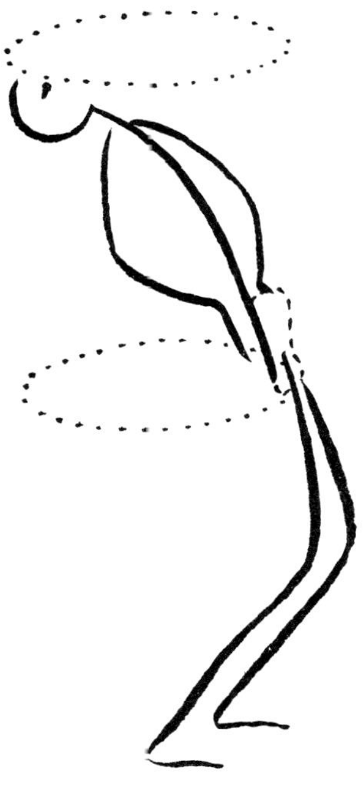

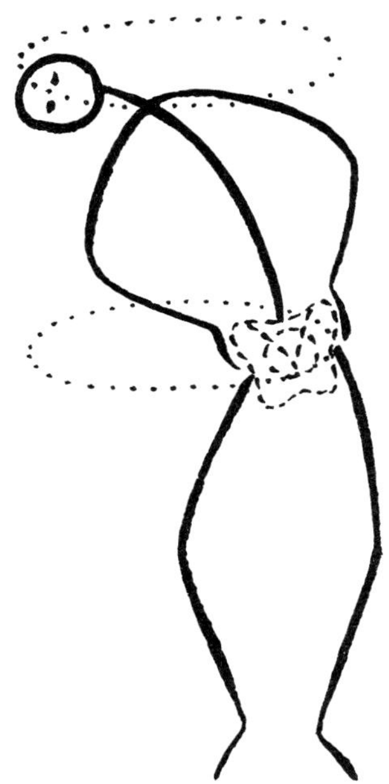

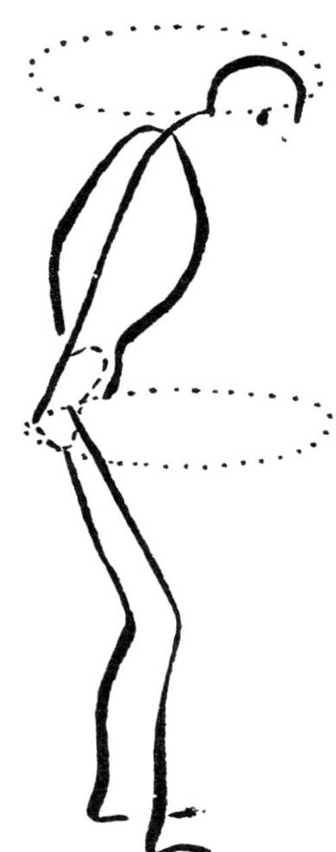

4. Move pelvis and tailbone forward, drop head backward. Describe circles with top of head and tailbone in opposite directions. When pelvis moves to right, head moves left; when pelvis moves backward, head moves forward; and so on.

Look at the sequence of drawings below. The centre of the hour-glass is the pivot point of the inverse cones in the mid-spine of the body which remains in a relatively fixed position. As the pelvis and head swing in opposite directions but with unified harmony, so the circumferences and edges of the cones rotate in exactly opposite directions, so that the sand flows from top to bottom in the same pattern as the empty space flows from bottom to top of the hour-glass.

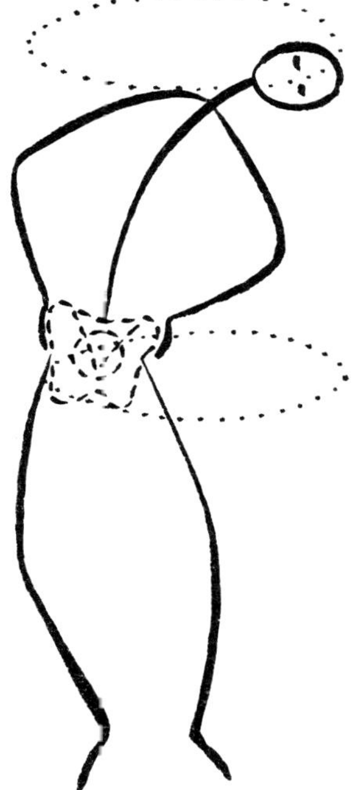

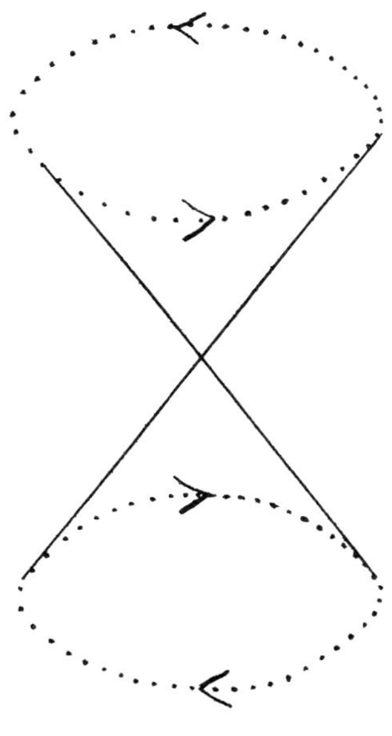

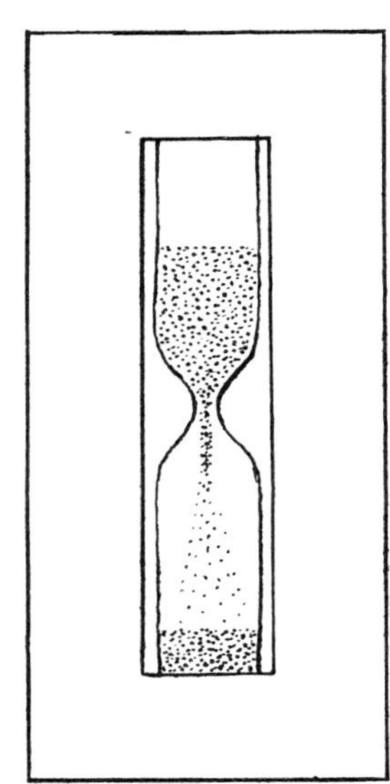

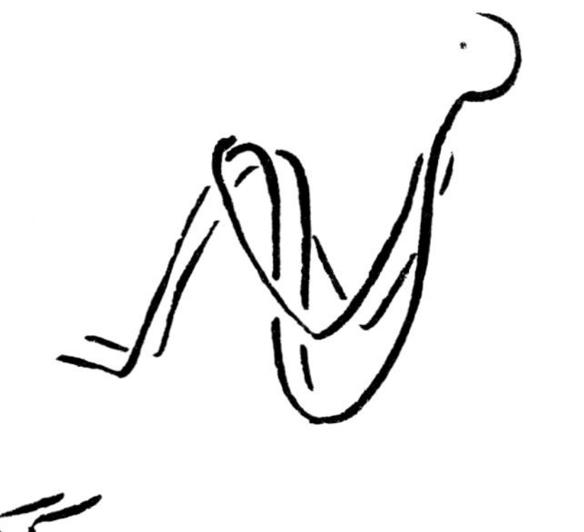

EXERCISE XXII

1. Sit on floor, legs together. Pull knees toward chest. Feet and hands off floor. Balance on tailbone.

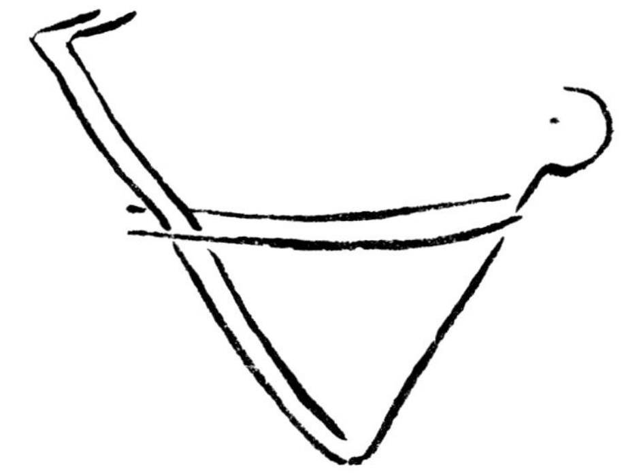

2. Straighten legs and stretch them upward while stretching arms forward. Feet should be higher than the head, knees between hands. Hands are at shoulder height, palms facing inward. Hold.

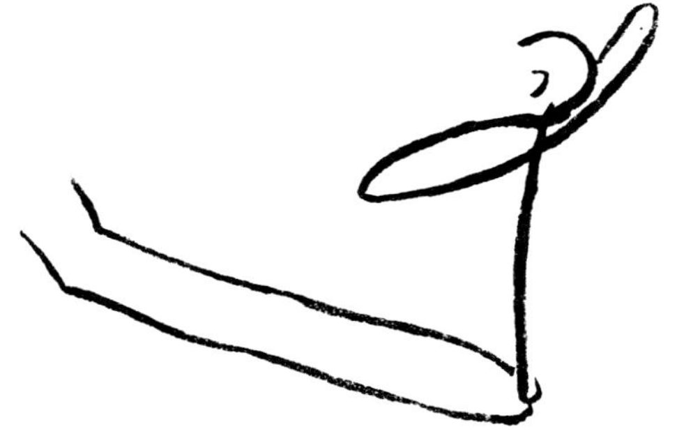

EXERCISE XXIII

1. Return to sitting position, legs straight and together. Interlace fingers behind base of skull.

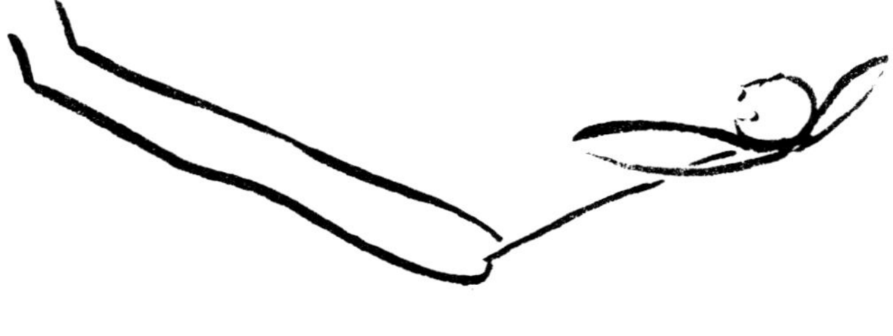

2. Lean backward as far as possible.

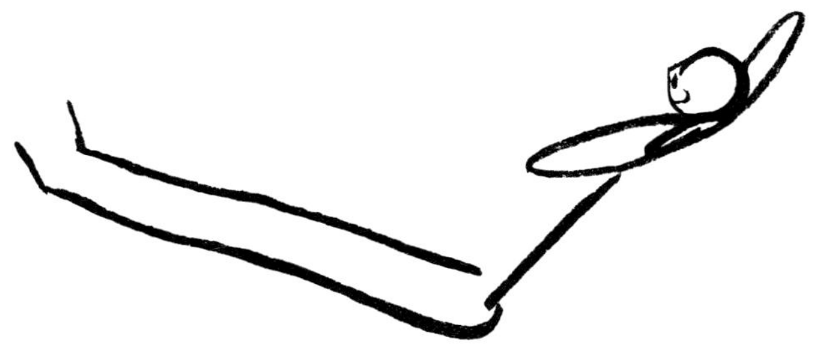

3. Now raise legs a foot above floor. Balance and hold.

EXERCISE XXIV

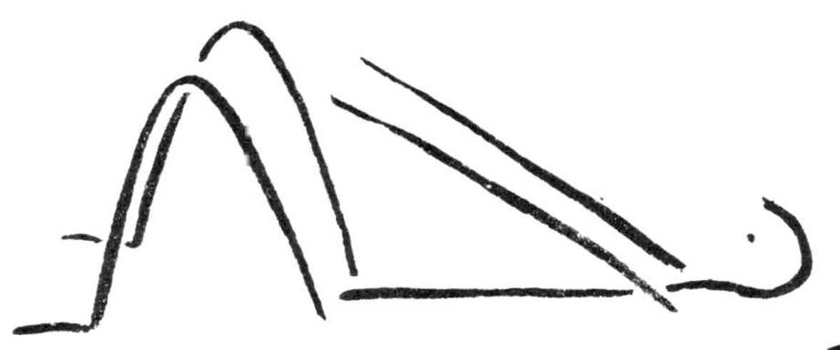

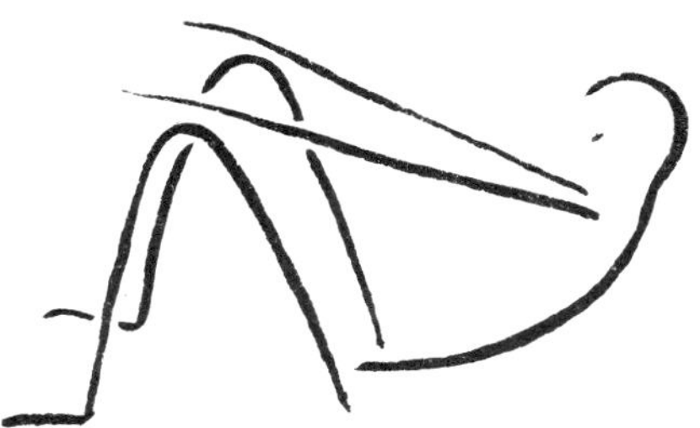

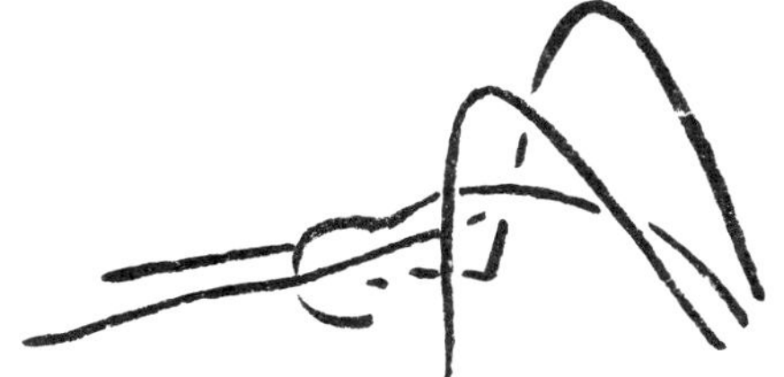

1. Lie down on back. Bend knees, placing feet one foot apart on floor. Arms stretch toward knees.

2. Lift spine off floor as much as possible. Stretch both hands to touch or reach beyond knees. Lie back down and come up many times.

3. Come up sitting and bend forward, reaching between knees as much as possible. Lie back down and come up. Repeat many times.

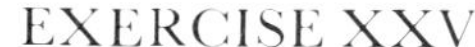

EXERCISE XXV

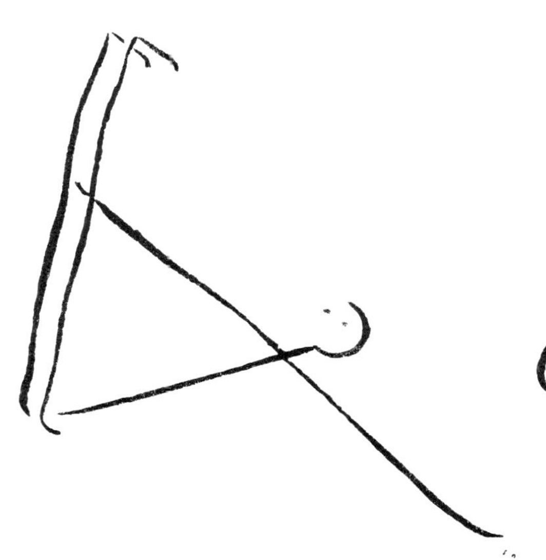

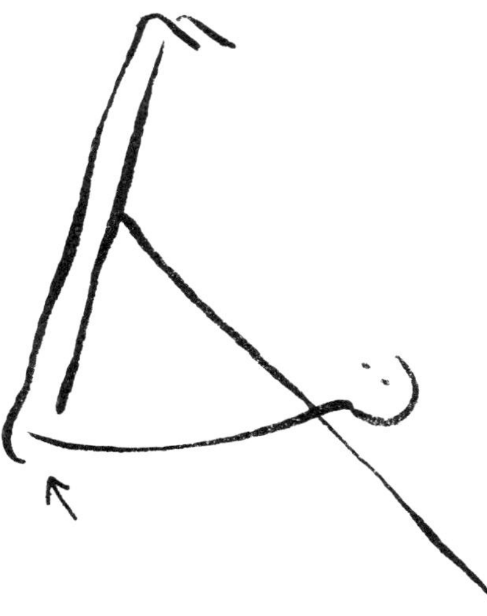

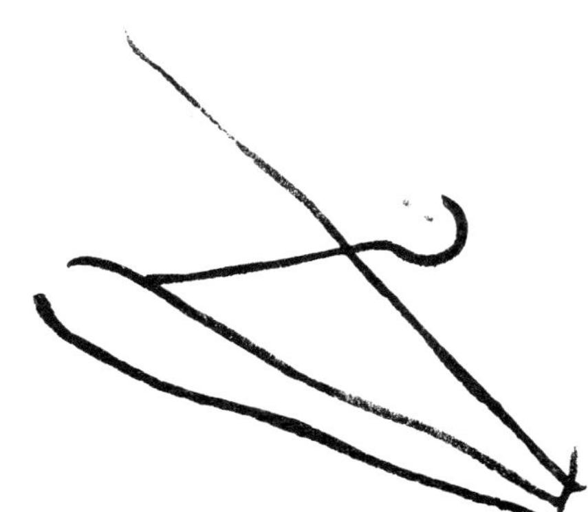

1. Lie on back, legs together, arms spread sideways. Palms up. Stretch both legs up straight.

2. Shift hips two inches to the right. Feet now point toward left hand.

3. Keeping legs straight, bring both feet down to touch left hand. Right shoulder remains on floor. Bring both legs back up together. Repeat several times. Repeat on other side.

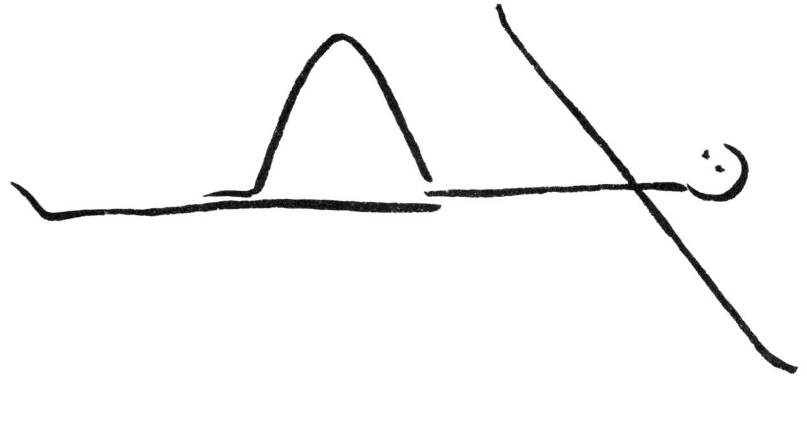

EXERCISE XXVI

1. Lie down on back, arms stretched sideways, palms up. Place right foot on top of left knee.

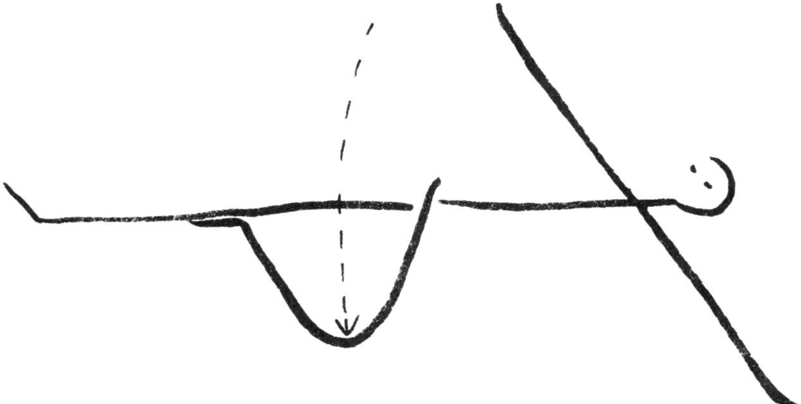

2. Move right knee toward left to touch floor. Right arm and shoulder may come off floor at first. Relax and let gravity gradually pull them toward floor. Hold. Bring knee up again and repeat with other leg.

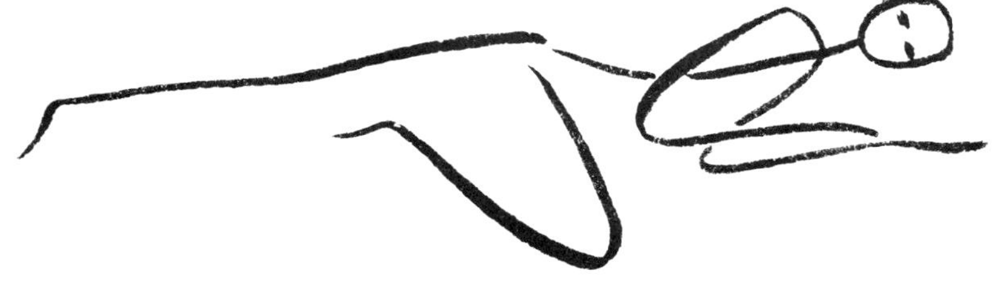

EXERCISE XXVII

1. Lie down on left side. Pull left knee up, so that thigh forms right angle with trunk.

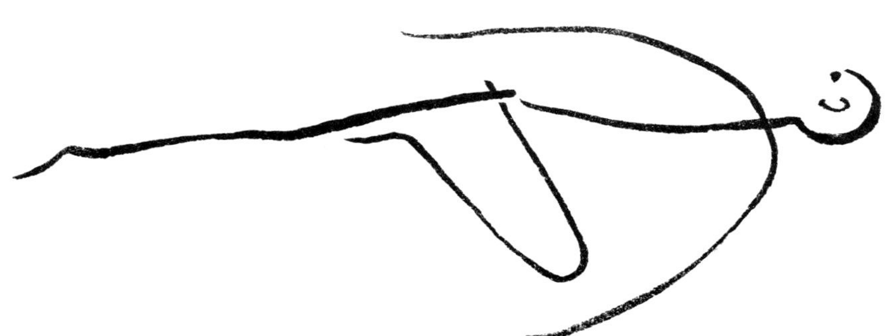

2. Place chest flat on floor. Place right cheek on floor. Both shoulders rest on floor, arms next to body. Relax any length of time in this position. Come up, roll on right side and repeat.

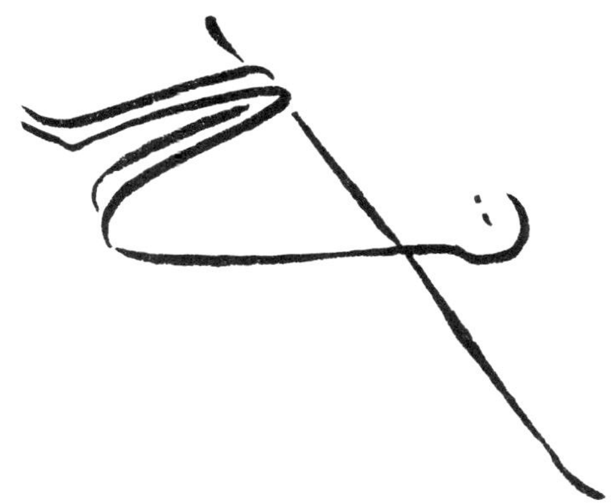

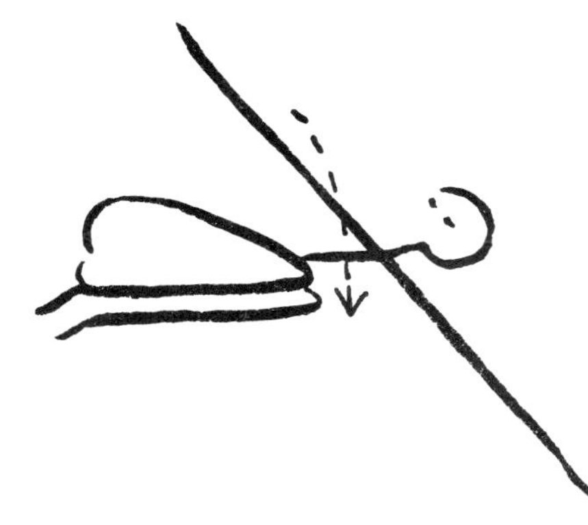

EXERCISE XXVIII

1. Lie down on back, legs together, arms stretched sideways. Pull knees toward chest.
2. Move knees and feet toward left, to touch floor. Keep left shoulder on floor. Keeping knees pulled up, raise and move them toward floor to the right. Repeat 20 times.

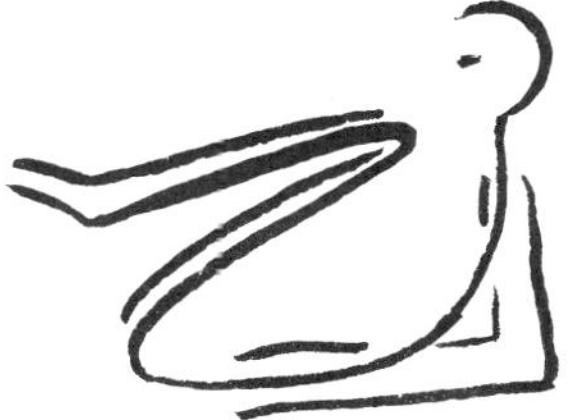

EXERCISE XXIX

1. Lie down. Lean back on elbows, palms flat on floor. Pull both knees up toward chest. Lower back rests on floor.

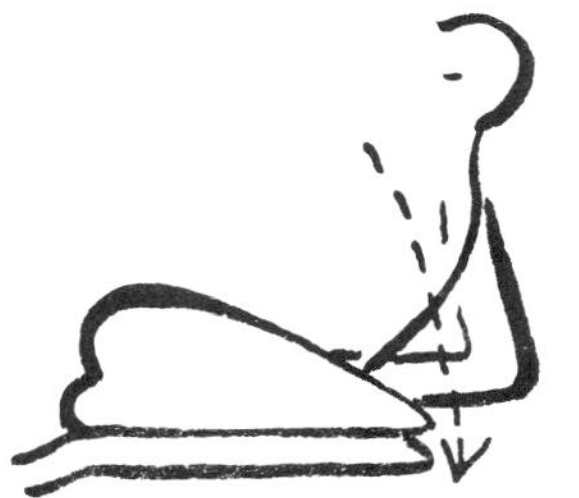

2. Keeping knees pulled high up, move knees and feet to left toward floor. Right hip and side of back come off floor. Keep both elbows in place, knees together. Do not strain. Bring knees back up to chest and move them toward the right. Repeat 20 times.

EXERCISE XXX

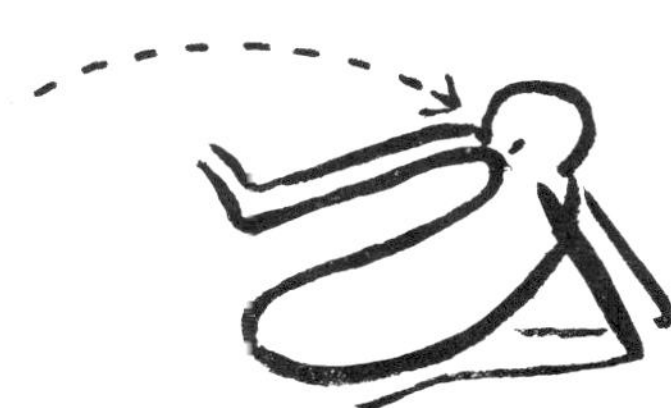

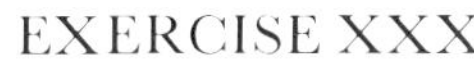

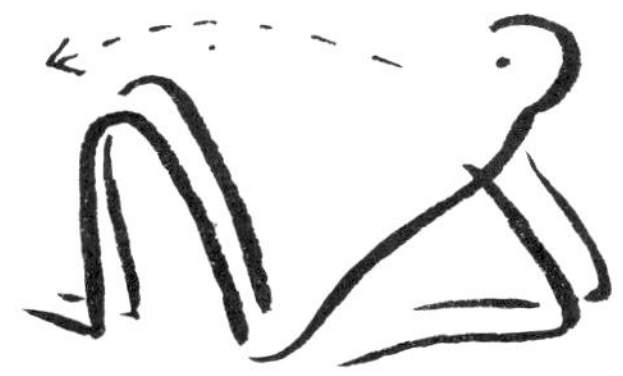

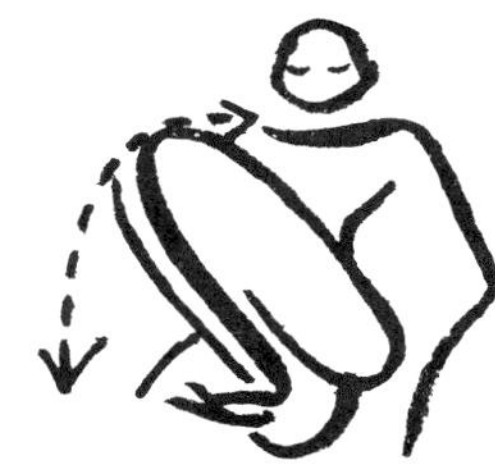

1. Pull knees up toward forehead. Lower back contacts floor. Knees and feet together.
2. Arch back and move pelvis foreward. Knees move away from face. Feet hang one inch above floor. Sitting bones and tailbone contact floor. Rock pelvis forward and backward, hollowing and rounding spine. Repeat many times.
3. Twist spine, so that feet and knees move to right. Only right part of hip rests on floor. Left knee moves toward right shoulder and then away. Repeat forward and backward rocking movement. Repeat on left side. An excellent exercise for lumbar vertebrae and massage of buttocks and hips.

EXERCISE XXXI

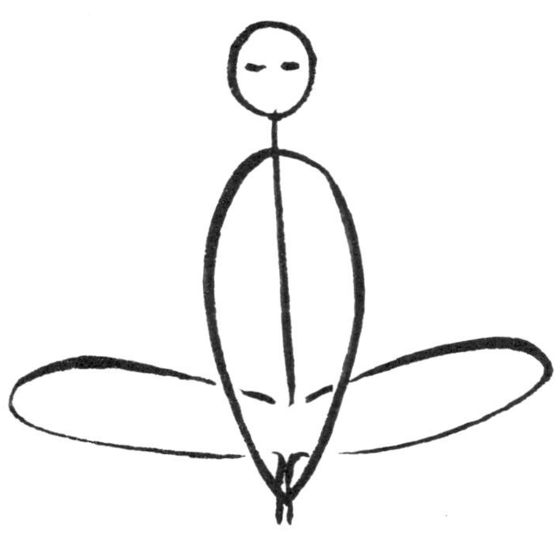

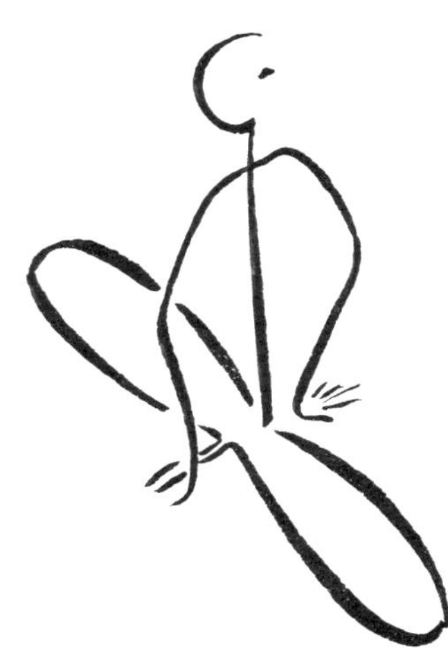

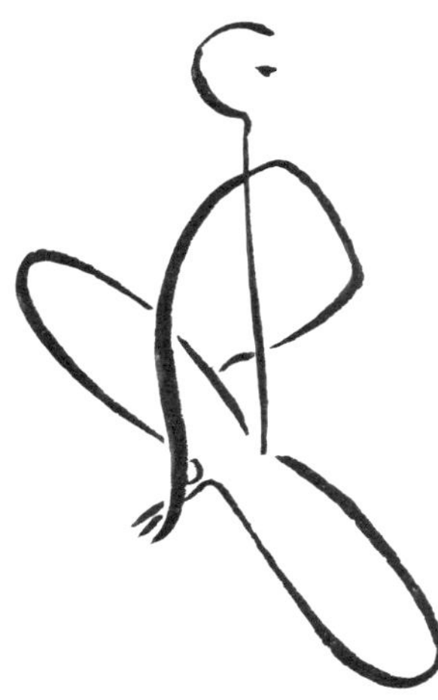

1. Sit in the tailor position.

2. Place left hand on floor behind tailbone and push against floor, so that spine straightens. Chestbone moves up. Right hand rests on top of left foot and pushes against foot, so that chest faces toward left. Left shoulder moves backward, right shoulder moves forward. Look over left shoulder. Release and repeat on other side.

3. If spine is straight, place back of left hand against back and repeat.

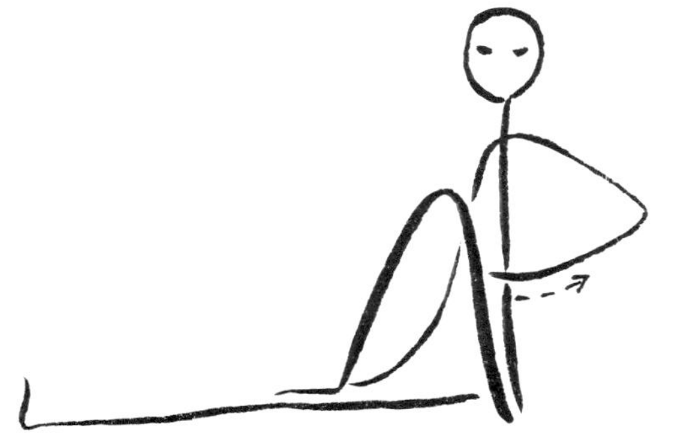

EXERCISE XXXII

1. Sit on floor. Spine and legs straight. Bring left foot over right leg and place it next to outside of right knee. Pull left thigh as close in as possible to abdomen and chest. Left knee moves toward right armpit. Left hand pulls stomach muscles to left. Chest faces left. Keep spine straight; raise chestbone.

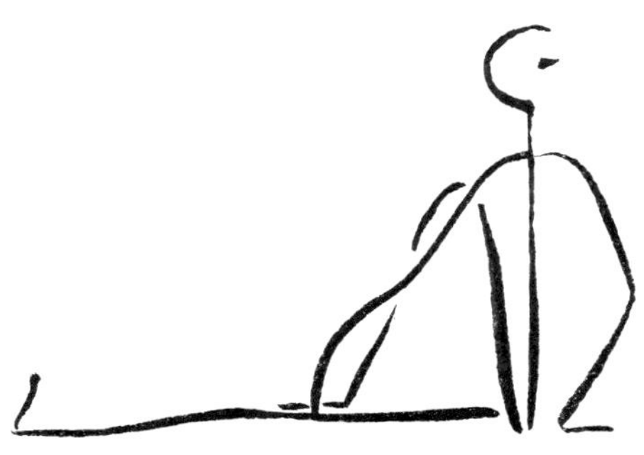

2. Move right arm so that upper arm touches outside of left knee. Right hand holds inside of left foot. Place left hand on floor behind tailbone. Push against floor so that spine straightens. Twist spine and look backward over left shoulder.

3. If spine is straight, place back of left hand against back. Left shoulder and chin move downward; base of skull moves upward. Stretch spine, while twisting from tailbone to base of skull. Right arm pushes slightly against left knee, so as to increase the twist. Repeat on other side.

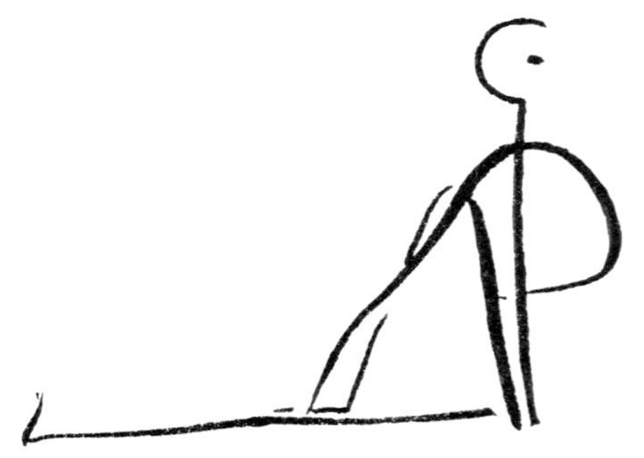

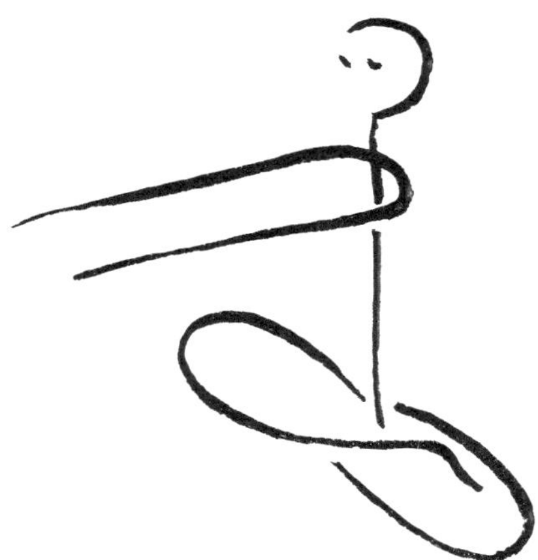

EXERCISE XXXIII

1. Sit in a comfortable position. Raise arms and bring them in front of body, hands in line with shoulders. Spine straight.

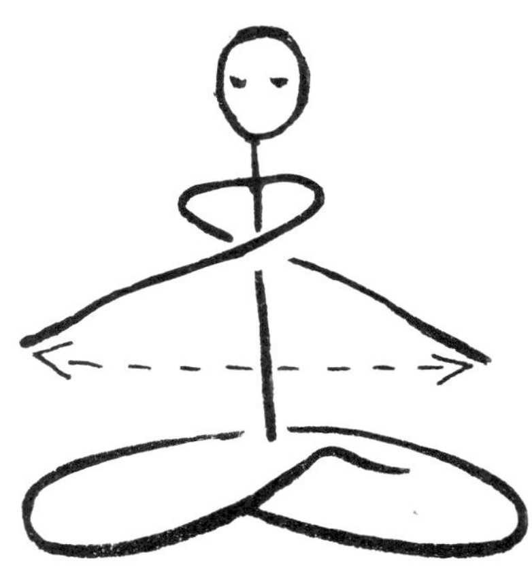

2. Keeping arms straight, move right arm to the left and left arm to the right. Alternate bringing one arm over the other. Repeat many times.

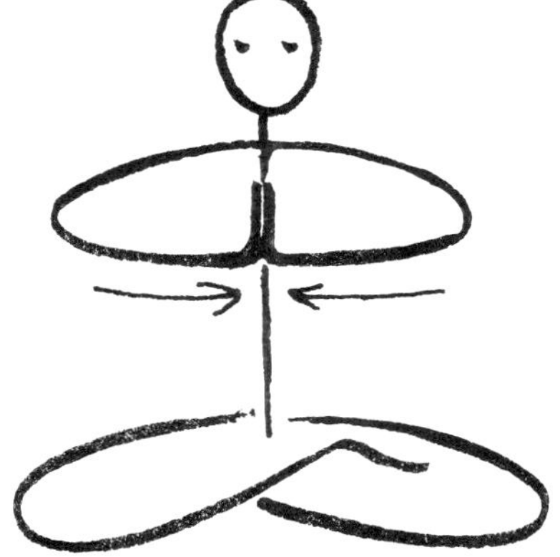

3. Bring palms together in front of chestbone. Press them together firmly for five counts. Relax and press again. Keep spine straight.
Repeat many times.

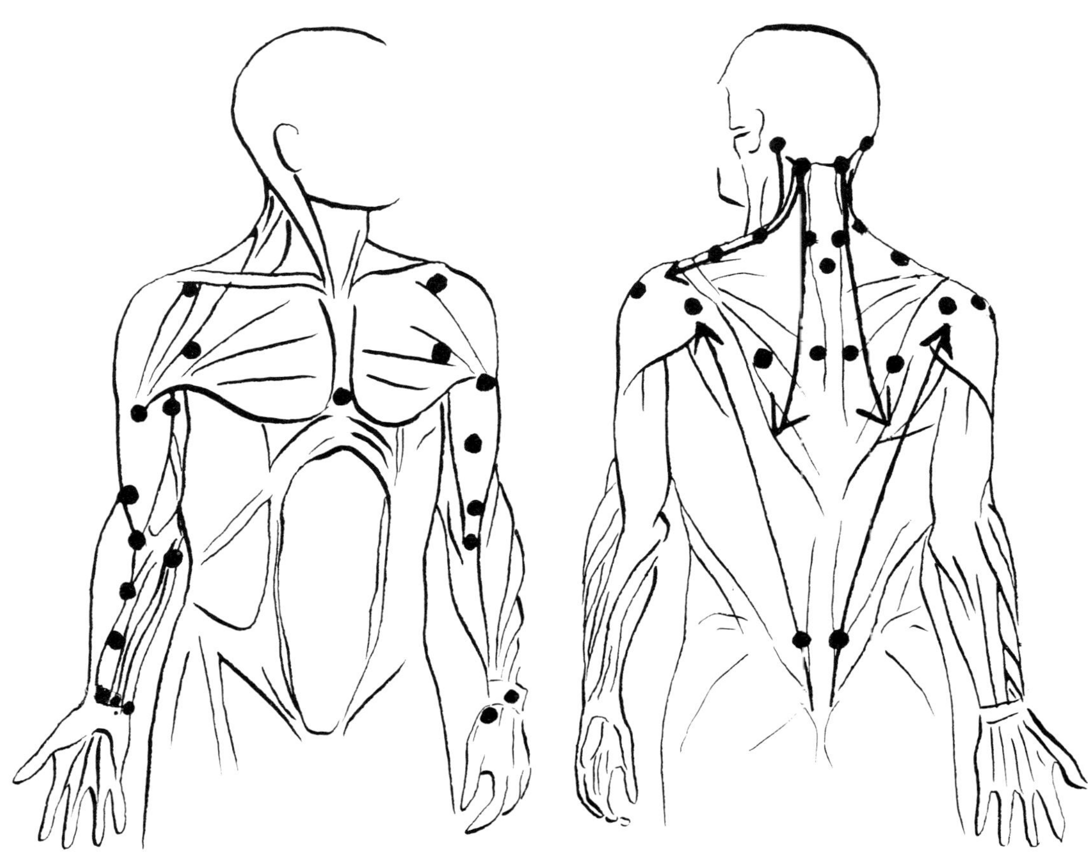

7. NECK, SHOULDERS AND ARMS

It is not by accident that the first vertebra (see p. 48) is called the atlas. Just as Atlas in the myth supported the burden of the earth on his neck and shoulders, so we carry our 'burden' around. If you look closely at people around you, perhaps you can see traces of bent upper backs, necks, and shoulders causing the head to tilt slightly forward or to the side. In this position the lungs are unable to breathe properly. Instead of the spine holding the topmost part of the body erect, the 'burden' weighs us down. We have to waste muscle power to perform the work of the skeletal system. So, again, the connection between the physical and psychological realms becomes apparent.

The neck area contains the throat as well as the beginning of the spine and spinal cord. The first exercise in this chapter co-ordinates breathing and vocal cord awareness. Tension in the neck will produce a tense, hoarse, or weak voice. Good posture, proper breathing, and strong voice all work together. Tension in the neck will also create tension in the eyes, as numerous nerves from both the central and autonomic systems connect the two areas. The exercise on p. 98 gives you a definite feeling for the interaction of head, eyes, neck, shoulders, arms, and trunk.

From the spinal cord in the neck, three major nerves enter and run the length of the arm. The arms are connected to the main skeleton by the collar-bones joining the spine at the base of the neck and the ball and socket joints connecting with the shoulder blades. The elbows are hinge joints; the wrists are gliding joints. (Note similarities to the structure of the leg.) Straighten and move your arm in as many directions as possible: one arm at a time, both arms together. Swing the arms backward and forward. Now repeat with one elbow bent, then the other, then with both elbows bent. Now straighten arm again, bend at wrist only; and repeat movements. Bend elbow and wrist together. Then shake the entire arm, allowing shoulder, elbow, and wrist joints to move as freely as possible. You may find it beneficial to perform this loosening up exercise before and/or after doing other exercises in this chapter. For the shoulderstand, elbowstand, handstand and headstand, which demonstrate the potential strength of the arms, see Chapter 10, 'Balance'.

7. Neck, Shoulders and Arms

EXERCISE I: AWARENESS OF THE VOICE

Lie down on your back and relax. Move awareness to your breathing without changing rhythm. Measure your inspiration and expiration times. Perhaps a partner could help you.

1. Now, open mouth and make a low ringing 'aah' sound while exhaling slowly. Sing the lowest sound you can make without strain. Continue with relaxed throat for one minute.
2. Keeping neck relaxed, roll head from right to left. Again make the low 'aah' sound. Continue for one minute and observe how head movement affects sound production.
3. Now, while moving head to the left, close right nostril with right thumb; and when head rolls to the right, close left nostril with right index finger. Continue for another minute, while making the low 'aah' sound, and observe how this affects quality of the sound.

Relax neck and head. Move awareness to breathing and repeat steps 1, 2, and 3 while singing the highest sound you can make without strain.

Relax again. Then repeat steps 1, 2, and 3 with mouth closed, making lowest possible humming sound. Then repeat 1, 2, and 3 while making highest possible humming sound without strain.

Then open your mouth again, make low 'aah' sound and slide up to highest sound you can produce and back down again. Repeat while rolling head for one minute. Keep body relaxed and observe whether it is easier to move from a low sound up or vice versa. Relax and move awareness to your breathing. Again measure inhaling and exhaling times.

EXERCISE II

1. Sit in relaxed or easy position. Spine straight. Arms relaxed. Drop head to the right and let it hang. Relax neck.

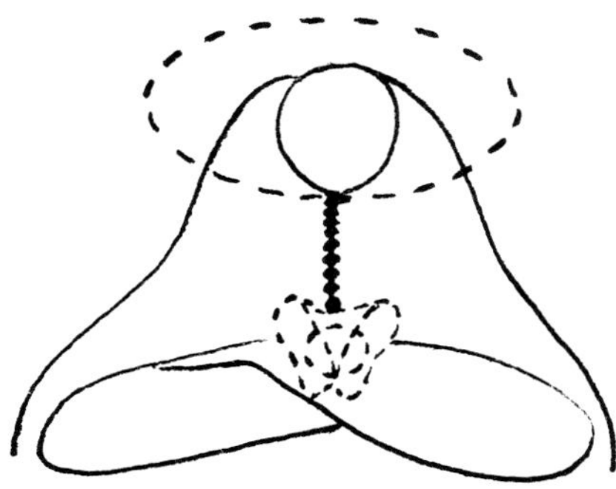

2. By moving trunk slightly forward, led head roll in forward hanging position. Without using neck muscles, roll head toward left shoulder. With a slight effort of the neck muscles, roll head over shoulder.

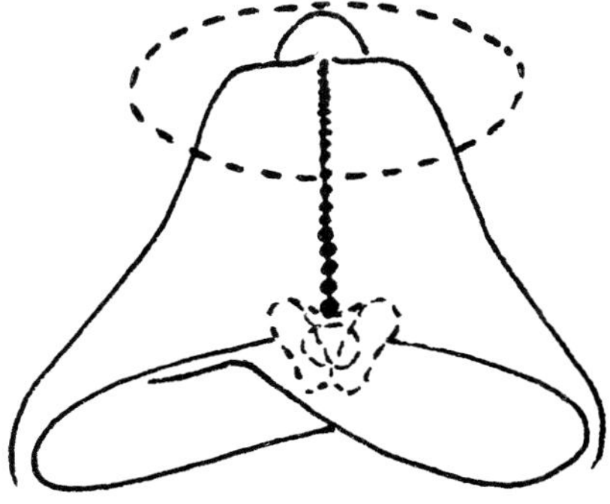

3. Drop head backward. Move head round in a circle by moving trunk and keeping neck muscles completely relaxed, clockwise and anti-clockwise.

7. Neck, Shoulders and Arms

EXERCISE III

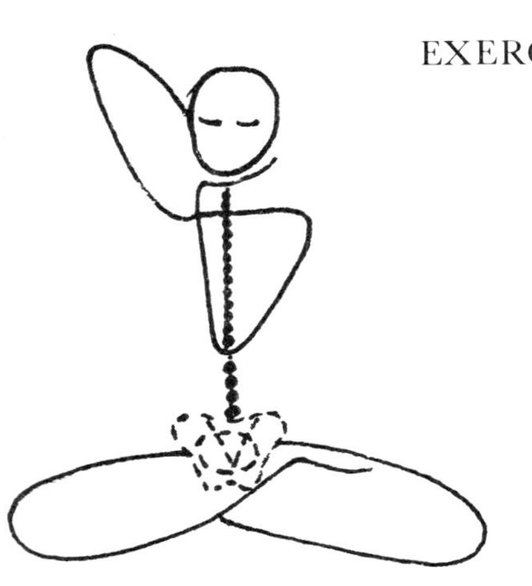

1. Place palm of left hand on right jawbone. Curl fingers under and around chin. Put right hand on base of skull. Keep chin slightly tucked in.

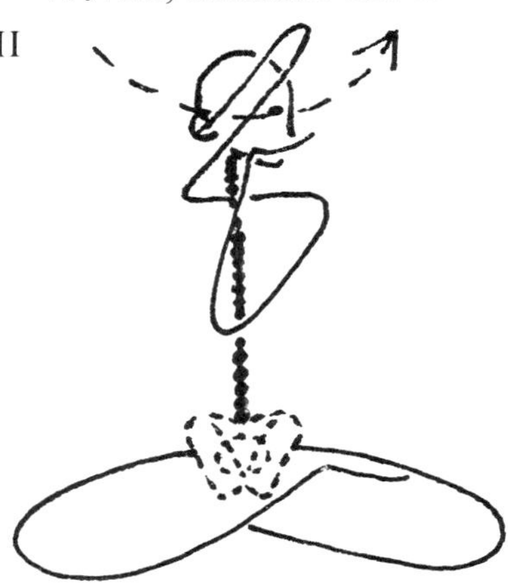

2. While pushing chin toward left shoulder with left hand, pull back of head forward with right hand. If you hold the hair, you will have a better grip. Neck may crack if it is sufficiently relaxed, but do not arch the neck. Repeat on other side.

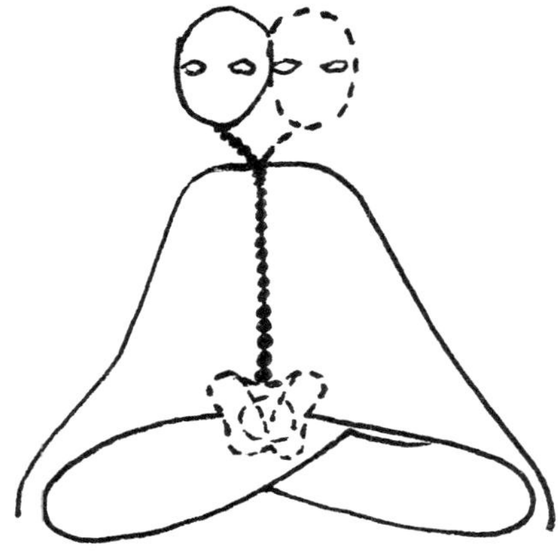

3. Look forward. Move left jawbone to left and then right jawbone to right. Head should not tilt sideways. Remain facing forward.

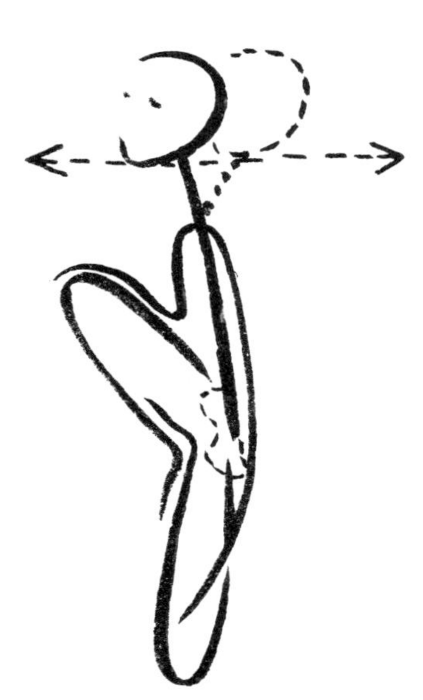

4. Move chin forward and backward. Avoid moving chin up and down. It may be useful to practice some of these exercises in front of a mirror.

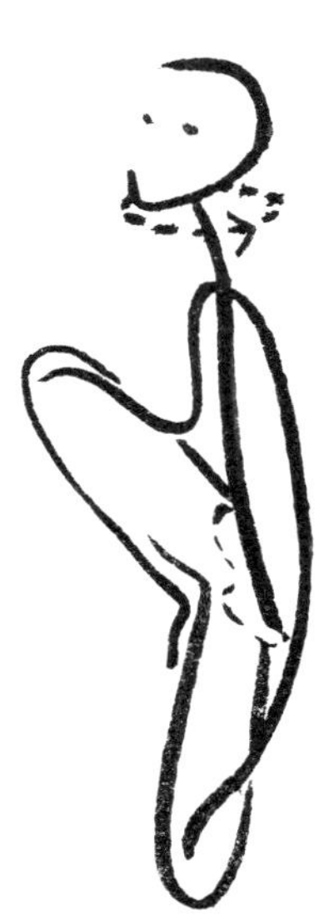

5. Facing forward, move chin to the left, forward, to the right, and backward, so as to describe a horizontal circle, clockwise and anti-clockwise.

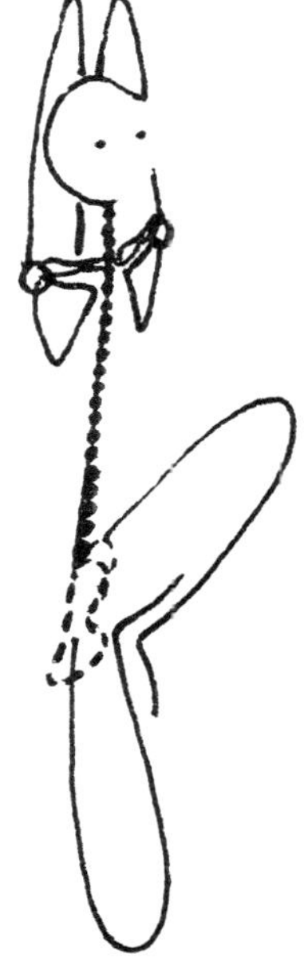

6. Stretch both arms upward. Place hands, one on top of the other, on upper part of spine, between shoulderblades. Elbows tuck behind back of head.

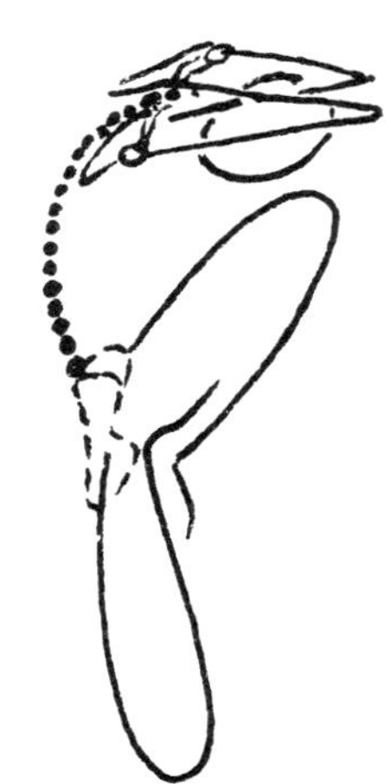

7. Press elbows against back of head to push chin against chestbone. Hold and gradually increase pressure on neck and upper spine.

EXERCISE IV

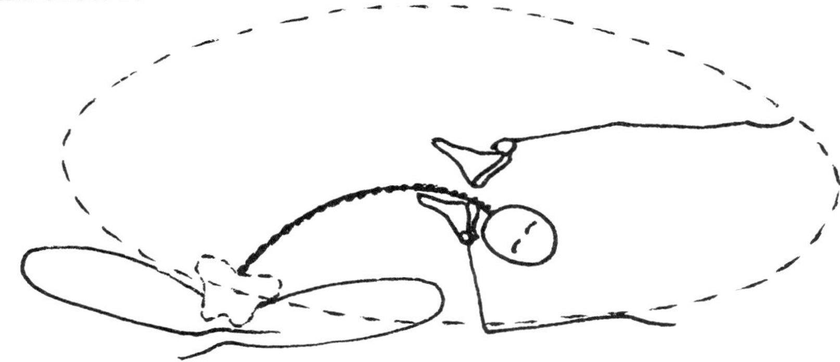

Sit in easy position. Lean to right and place right elbow on floor, about one foot away from right hip, palm on floor. Stretch left arm upward. Describe a large circle around you with left arm. Reach as far forward, backward, and sideways as possible, keeping arm straight. Repeat many times, clockwise. and anti-clockwise, first slowly, then as fast as possible. Movement comes from left shoulder joint. Repeat on other side.

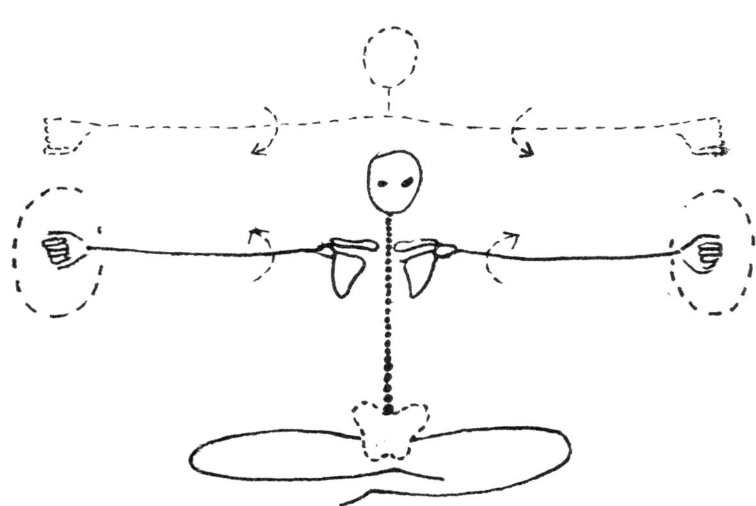

EXERCISE V

1. Hold arms out sideways. Then rotate arms from shoulder joint, so that top of hands face wall in front of you. Continue rotation as far as comfortable.
   Then reverse direction so that wrist, fist, and arm move in direction of wall in front of you. Top of hand should face floor or continue even further if rotation is comfortable. Repeat movements many times.

2. Then turn right fist downward and left fist up. Each time fists turn, move head toward fist that moves upward. Repeat many times. Then turn face toward fist that moves downward. Repeat many times.

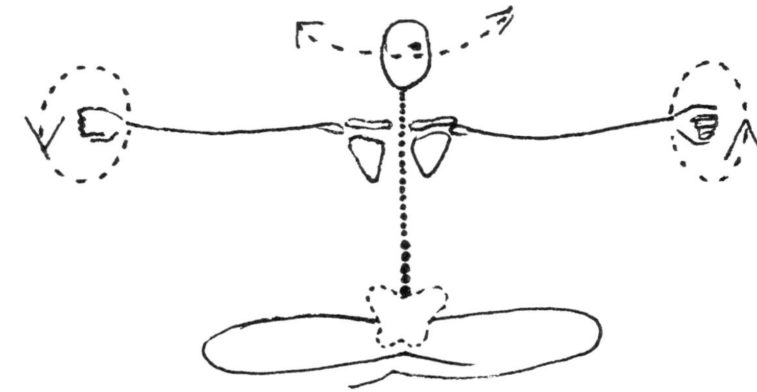

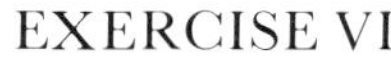

EXERCISE VI

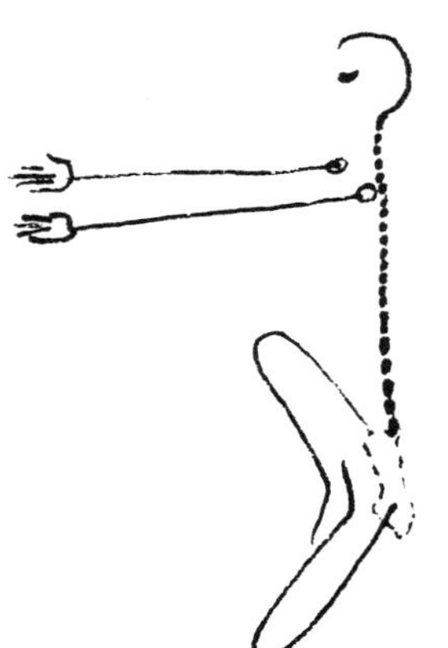

. Sit in easy position.
Stretch both arms in front of you, parallel to floor, palms facing each other.

. Then turn palms outward and cross left arm over right.

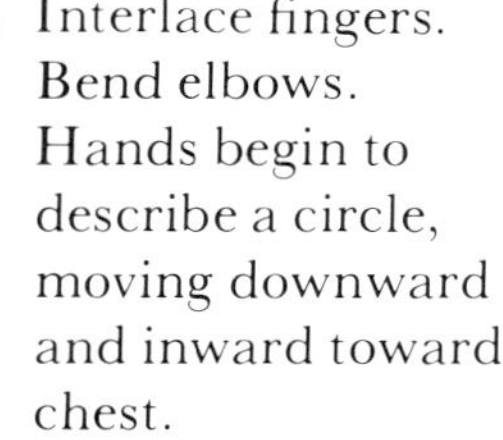

. Interlace fingers.
Bend elbows.
Hands begin to describe a circle, moving downward and inward toward chest.

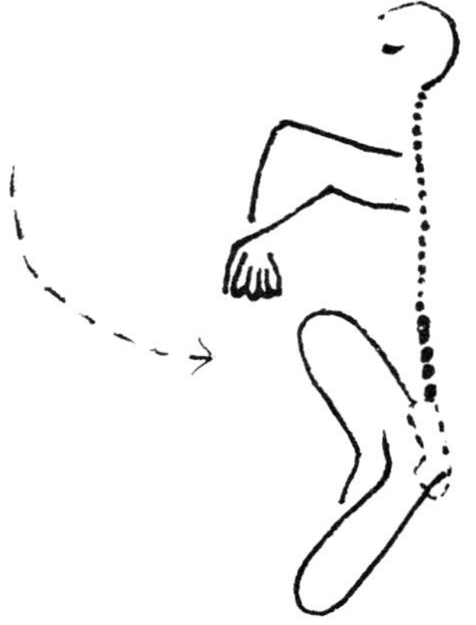

. Move hands further in and up toward face.
Stretch arms and move hands away from you.
Do not release grip.
Reverse circular motion and repeat three times. Then repeat with right arm crossed over left arm.

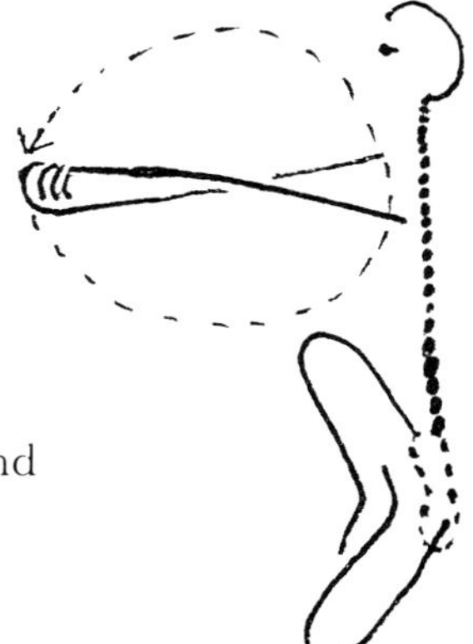

EXERCISE VII

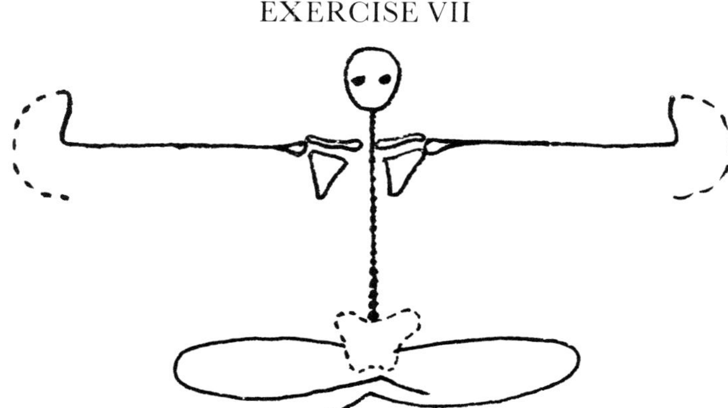

1. Now, stretch arms out horizontally, palms facing floor. Keeping hands and fingers straight, bend wrists and point fingers upward as far as possible, then downward as far as possible. Repeat many times.

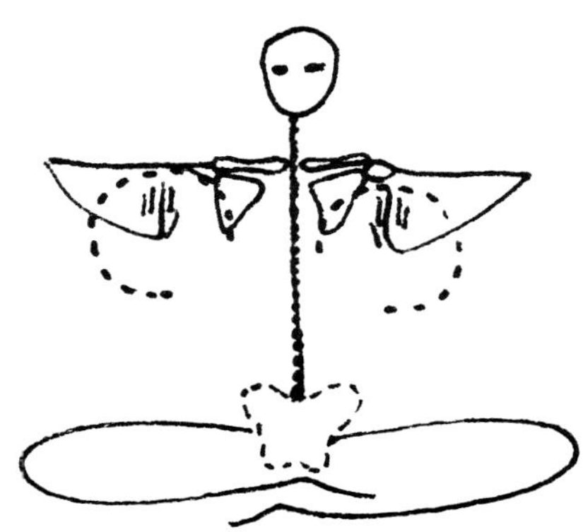

2. With arms outstretched and horizontal, bend elbows and bring hands in front of body, fingers pointing upward. Keeping palms facing forward, turn hands around in a semi-circular movement until fingers point downward. Then reverse movement. Repeat many times. Elbows remain at shoulder height.

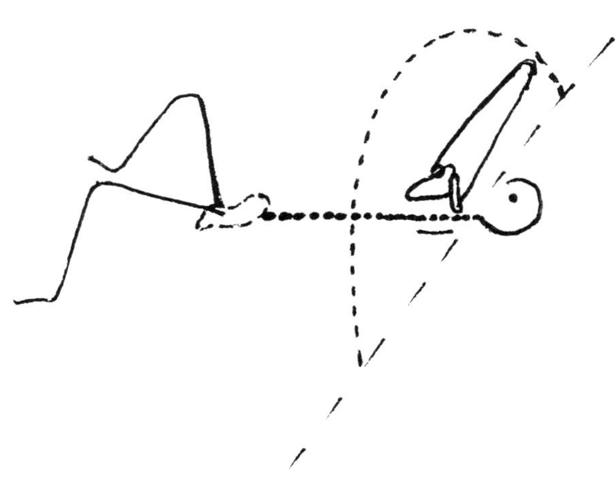

EXERCISE VIII

Lie down with feet wide apart, about two feet from body. Stretch both arms upward toward ceiling. Interlace fingers. Move hands and arms to the right toward floor. Hands do not necessarily contact floor. Keep arms straight and both buttocks on floor. Look upward. Left shoulderblade and upper back leave floor. Upper part of spine and shoulders should stay loose. Move arms from right to left many times.

EXERCISE IX

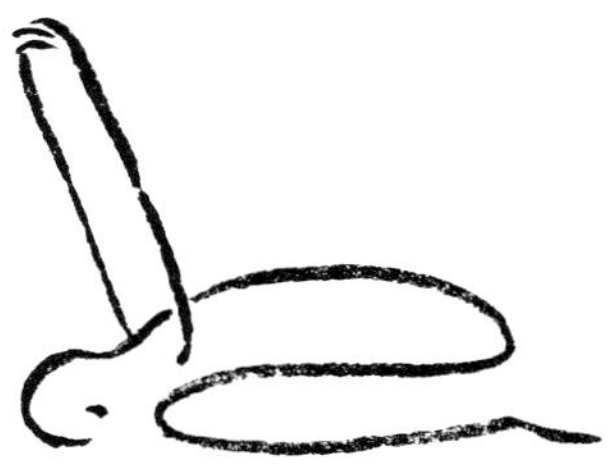

1. Kneel on floor. Sit back on heels. Rest forehead on floor. Interlock fingers behind back.

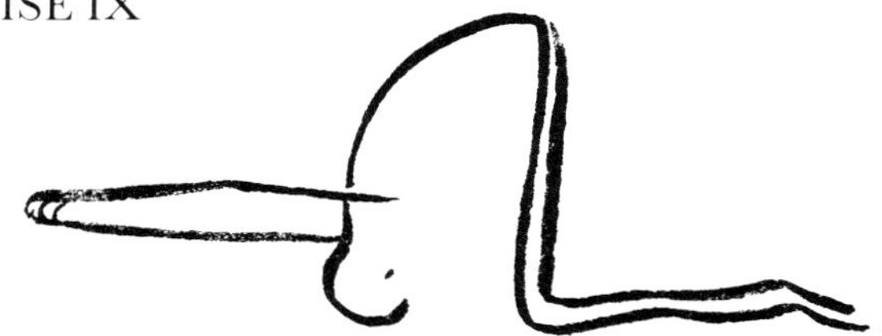

2. Come up on knees and roll forward, so that top of head rests on floor. The trunk is now supported by knees, head, and feet. Straighten arms and move hands over head toward floor. Relax and hold.

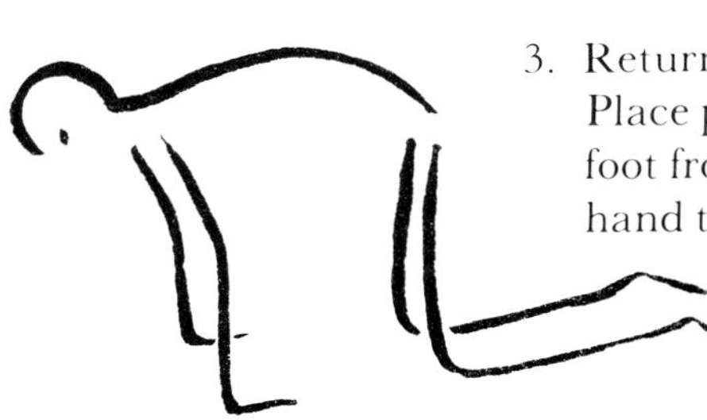

3. Return to kneeling position. Place palms on floor one foot from knees. Turn right hand to right, left hand to left until fingers point toward knees.

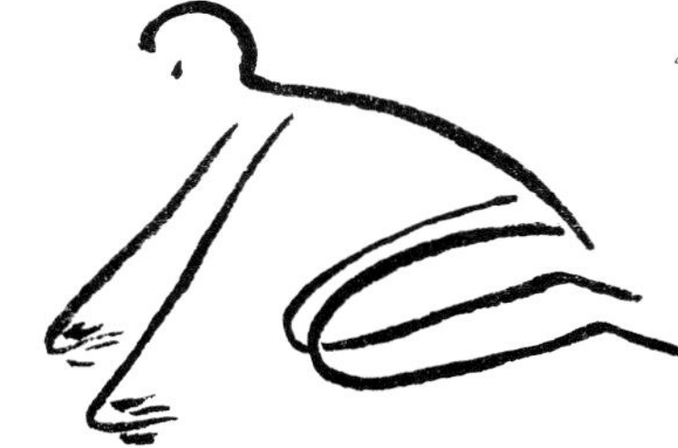

4. Dig balls of hands firmly into floor while sitting back on heels. Hold stretch as long as pleasant.

EXERCISE X

1. Stand with right foot two to three feet in front of left foot. Hang forward, chestbone over thigh. Avoid swinging toward left. Hold.

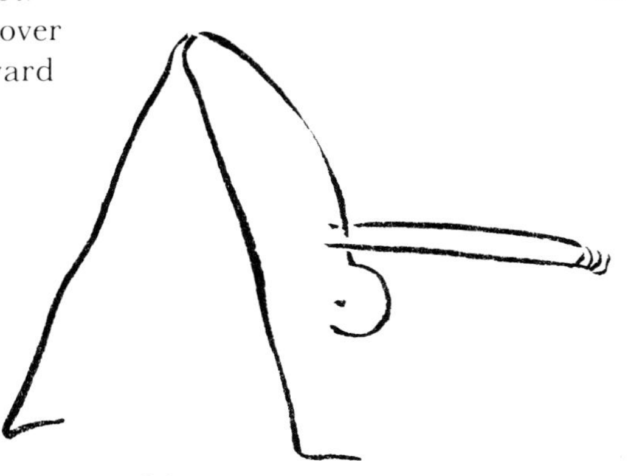

2. Interlace fingers behind back. Straighten arms, pull shoulders backward, shoulder blades together. Move arms upward and over head toward floor. Keep legs straight. Move hands toward floor with light bouncing movements. Come back up and repeat with other leg in front.

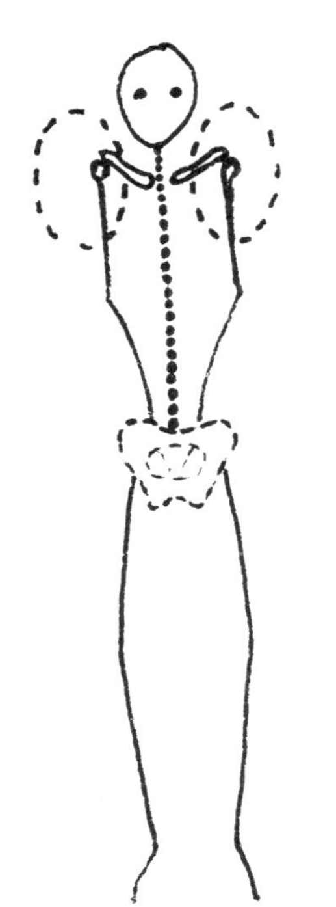

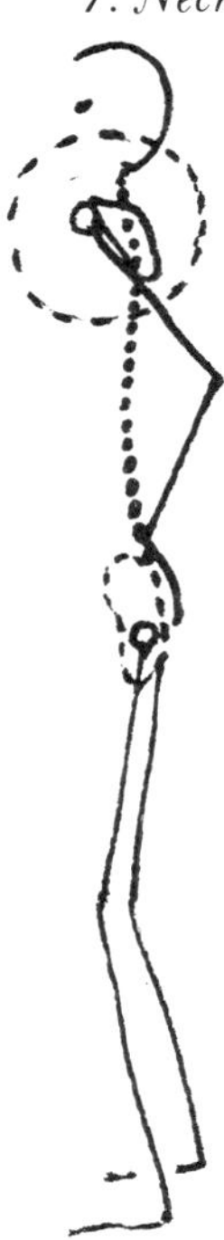

EXERCISE XI

Stand with feet one foot apart, toes pointed forward. Place hands on lower back, with edges of hands touching. Elbows move backward. Pull shoulders up towards ears, as high as possible. Move them forward, downward, backward, and up again, describing two circles, clockwise and anti-clockwise, fast and slow.
Then turn only one shoulder at a time, in both directions.
Relax arms and swing them loosely in circles, clockwise and anti-clockwise.

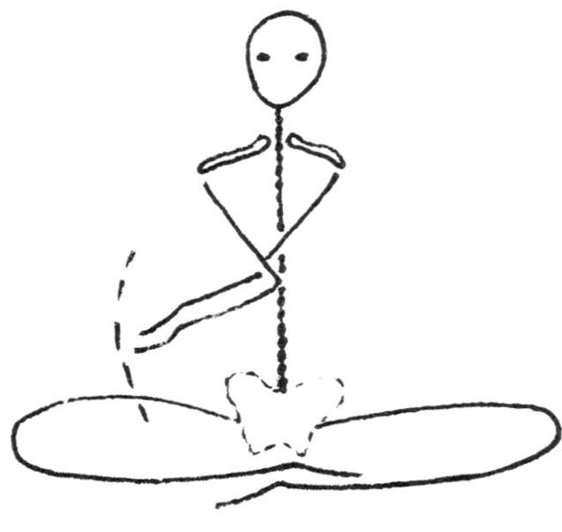

EXERCISE XII

Sit in easy position. Bring left arm in front of chest, bent slightly at elbow. Hook right elbow underneath left upper arm. Left palm facing upward, right palm downward. Move right hand toward left wrist and place palm on top of left wrist or hand. Right hand pushes left hand down. Left elbow is kept in a firm lock. Keep spine straight. Then gently bounce left hand down. Then pull it up, move it to the left, and bounce down gently. Repeat several times, then on other side of body.

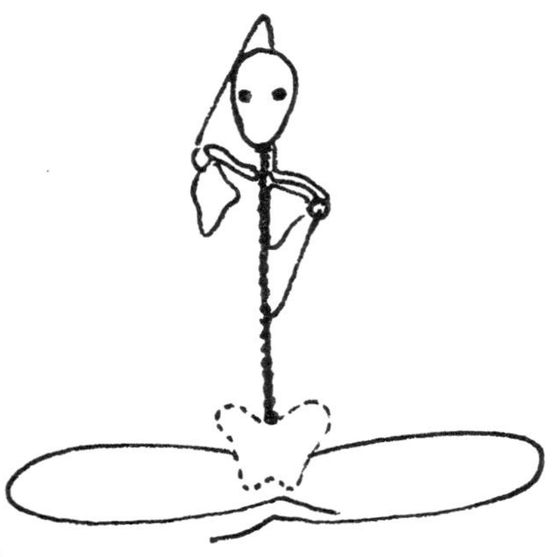

EXERCISE XIII

Sit in easy position. Place top of right hand against upper part of spine, as high as possible, fingers pointing upward. Stretch left arm upward, move left hand toward right hand, and hook fingers together. Elbows should be as much in line with spine as possible. Slowly increase grip. Hold. Release and repeat with other arm.

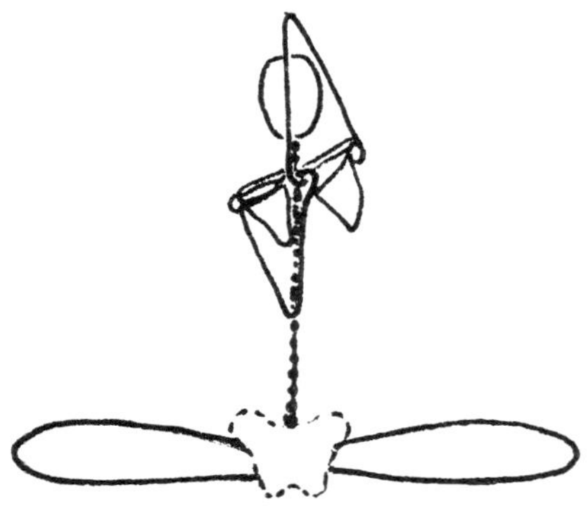

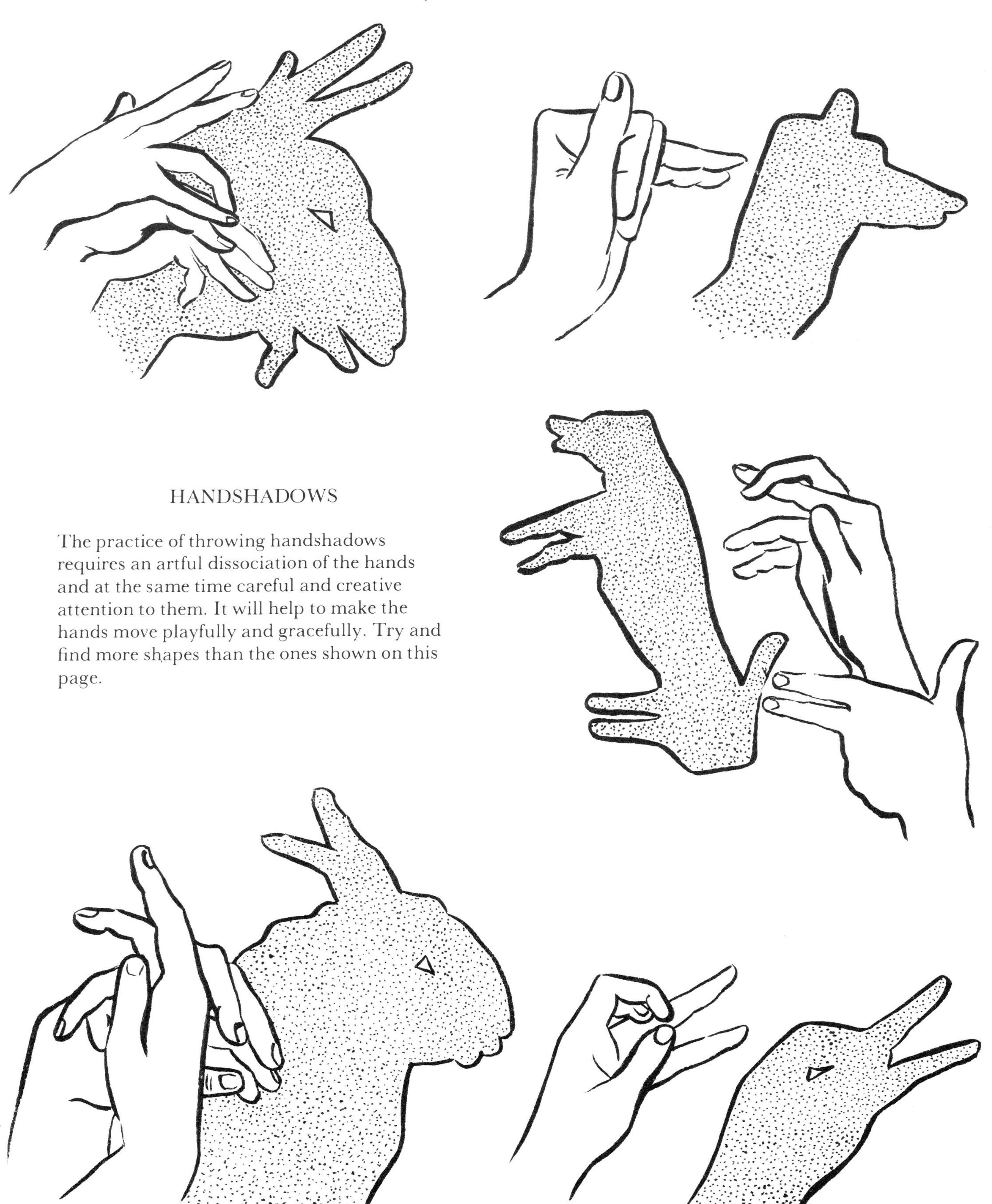

HANDSHADOWS

The practice of throwing handshadows requires an artful dissociation of the hands and at the same time careful and creative attention to them. It will help to make the hands move playfully and gracefully. Try and find more shapes than the ones shown on this page.

8. HEAD AND FACE

The skin of face and neck, unlike that of the rest of the body, is one with the muscles. When an emotion is experienced, the muscles and skin contract together, commanded by the facial nerves. Overactive nerves can cause twitches in different parts of the face, facial cramps, and even toothaches. People often speak of worry lines on their foreheads. The trigeminal nerves control the functions of mastication, perspiration, and crying. The pressure points shown in drawing on p. 97 are located on branches of the trigeminal nerves. Combined with the exercises that follow, regular massage of face and pressure points will keep face smooth, relaxed, and free of unnecessary wrinkles.

FACE MASSAGE

Begin by slapping your face with both hands, more and more vigorously, to stimulate nerves and blood circulation, and so removing blocks in the energy flow. Exhale freely. Use cold water or a face tonic to increase the revitalising effect of the massage. The fingers should slide smoothly over skin; so cover the whole face with cream or oil, rubbing it in with upward and outward stroking movements.

Take hold of tip of chin (pressure point 1) with tip of middle finger and thumb firmly tucked under chinbone. Massage deeply. Relax jaw muscles and open mouth by pushing chin downward with grip of finger and thumb. Open and close mouth many times, until jaw muscles have really relaxed. Then, with both hands simultaneously, move up along chin, pressing deeply towards points 2 at corner of mouth and 3 on side of chin. Dwell on spots that feel painful or tense. Continue along jaw toward ear. With deep circular movements, massage all around ear. Pinch and rub ear with index finger and thumb until ear is glowing. Pull it upward; push it forward against head; pull down the earlobes. Move to point 4 and massage with deep rotating movements. Then gently stroke in direction of arrow toward points 5 and 6. Then press lightly and rapidly with middle fingers and thumb on each side of esophagus down to thyroid gland at base of throat. Then dig fingers under jawbone, working out tender or lumpy spots. Press deeply into cheeks, lips, and jaws to stimulate gums. Return to point 1 and stroke upward over chin, mouth, and jaw toward ear.

Press on points 7 and 8, holding down for five seconds, then releasing. Repeat several times. Then stimulate cheekbones and side of nose with circular massage in direction of ears, resting at point 9. Massage this area with deep rotating movements. This is the area of the temporo-mandibular joint. Bad oral hygiene as a child – biting fingernails, sucking thumb and the like – can effect this joint and the adjacent muscle. Regular massage and jaw exercise can slowly ease this tension. Stroke left and right cheeks alternately to avoid stretching or pulling of skin. Open mouth and massage jaw muscles from inside! Place thumb of right hand inside left cheek, tips of index and middle fingers on outside of cheek. Dwell on hard and sensitive spots. Move backward to where jaw is attached to skull.

Pinch tip of nose. Then pinch bridge of nose and pull forward several times. With fingertip draw a line from tip of nose over forehead up to hairline. Repeat many times. Dwell on spot above nose between eyebrows, stroking upward and outward. Firmly press points 10, 11, 12, 13, and 14, massaging as indicated on diagram. For deeper relaxation of forehead, stroke with knuckles. Finally stroke in direction of arrows in long slow movements, wiping away all thoughts, memories, worries, and wrinkles.

Stimulate and relax top of head by hammering scalp gently with knuckles of both fists. Grab fistfuls of hair and pull firmly. Massage skull with fingertips as forcefully as you can.

Gently press palms of hands on eyes. Hold about ten seconds, then release pressure. Repeat five times.

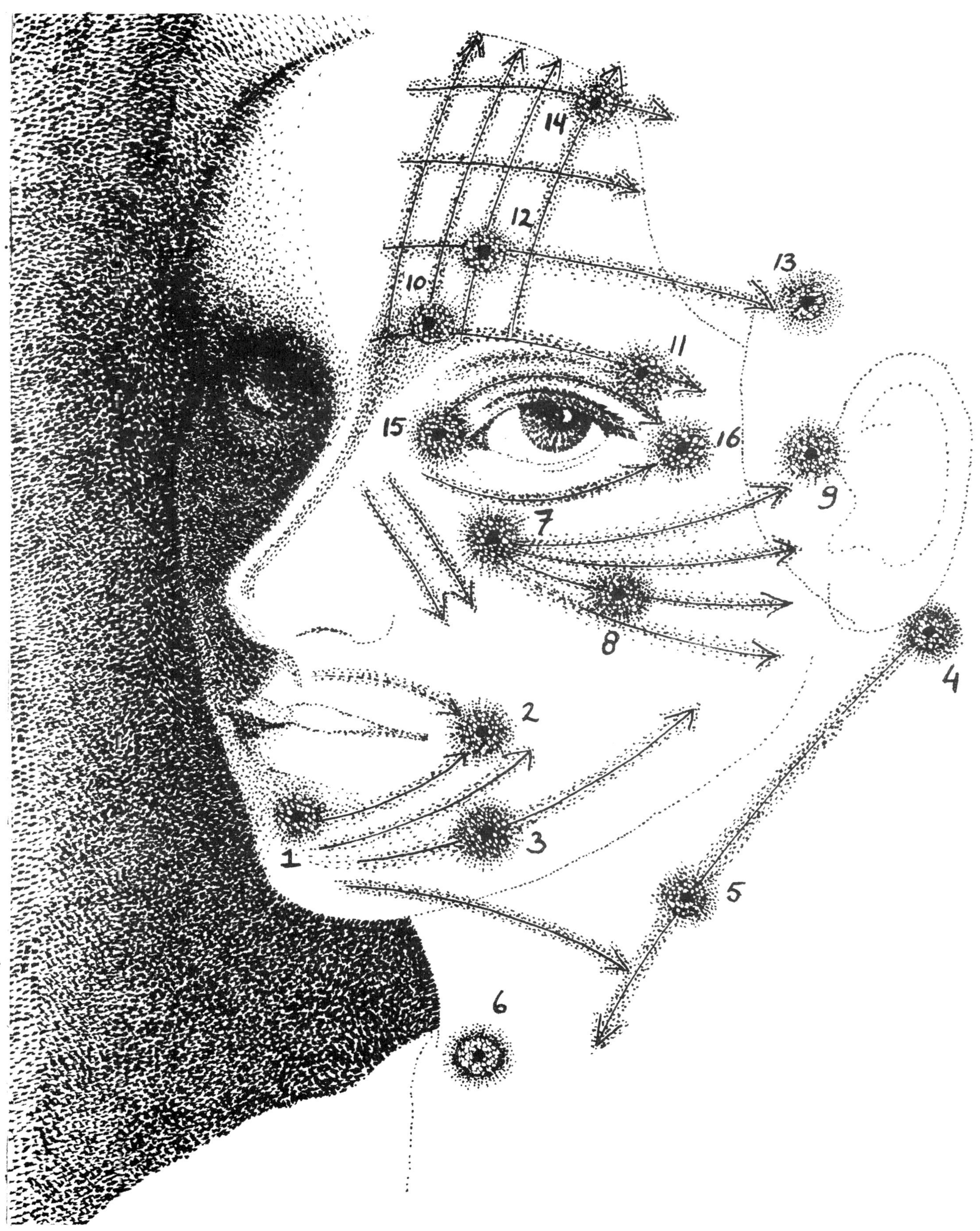
14
12
13
10
11
15
16
9
7
8
4
2
1
3
5
6

8. Head and Face

With a gentle raising and lowering of finger, move from point 15 to 16 over upper edge of eyeball. Repeat over lower edge of eyeball. Feeling should be pleasant. Then press gently around eye, exploring whole case of eye. Be subtle and gentle while tapping area on and around eye with light fast movements. Do not rub or pull on skin around eyes.

Finally, .splash face with cold water or a face tonic. Continue with exercises for the face, if you feel sufficiently invigorated. Massage and exercises work in tandem to increase your awareness and improve your health.

EXERCISE I: FACIAL EXERCISES

These exercises for jaw, mouth, tongue, cheeks, and eyebrows need not be practised in sequence. Perform them as often as and as long as comfortable.

Lie down on your back and relax, especially the jaw, so that your mouth is at least half open. Move lower jaw forward as far as possible and bring lower teeth in front of upper teeth, keeping mouth open. Hold a while; then pull jaw back in as far as possible. Repeat many times. Then move lower teeth in front of upper teeth and slowly move jaw all the way to the right, then to the left. Imagine a half circle in front of your face and make jaw travel over its outline, slowly without any jerks. Then open mouth as wide as possible and hold. Pull corners of mouth to ears and move lips forward to shape an O. Repeat many times and relax. Then curl lips backward. First open and curl them back with fingers; then try to hold them in position, using lip muscles only. Hold as long as possible.

Open your mouth and stick tongue out as far as possible. Stretch even further, try to reach your chin. Then stretch tongue upward to nose. Move it up and down several times. Now describe a circle with tip of tongue sliding over and around lips, clockwise and anti-clockwise. Repeat many times. Then move tip of tongue inside lips over gums, keeping lips closed. Move tongue slowly over upper gum line from left to right, returning along lower gum line from right to left. Push tip of tongue as far up (or down) gum line and as far back as possible. Repeat in other direction. After this series of exercises, get up and look in a mirror. The expression of your mouth will have changed, and your whole face will be looking much more relaxed.

Shape your mouth as if to make an O, an EE, and an AH sound. Repeat one after the other many times. Then pull right corner of mouth to the right. Repeat five times. Then move right corner to the left five times, keeping left corner of mouth relaxed. Repeat exercise with left corner of mouth. Then slowly move whole mouth from right to left.

Now open your mouth as if to make an AH sound, teeth about one inch apart. Though it is not possible, try to close lips without moving jaw. Nose will pull downward. Keep mouth in same position and place tips of thumb and index finger against nostrils to close them. Now try to open passage using nostril muscles to push fingers away.

Blow cheeks up like a balloon with lips closed. Then expel the air forcefully through a small opening. Immediately after, suck cheeks in as deep as possible. Repeat several times.

Raise both eyebrows and drop them. Repeat several times. Raise and drop one eyebrow at a time. Practise in front of a mirror. Now move eyes and eyebrows upward at the same angle. Then repeat with each eye individually. Then hold eyebrows in upward position and move eyes downward. Repeat several times.

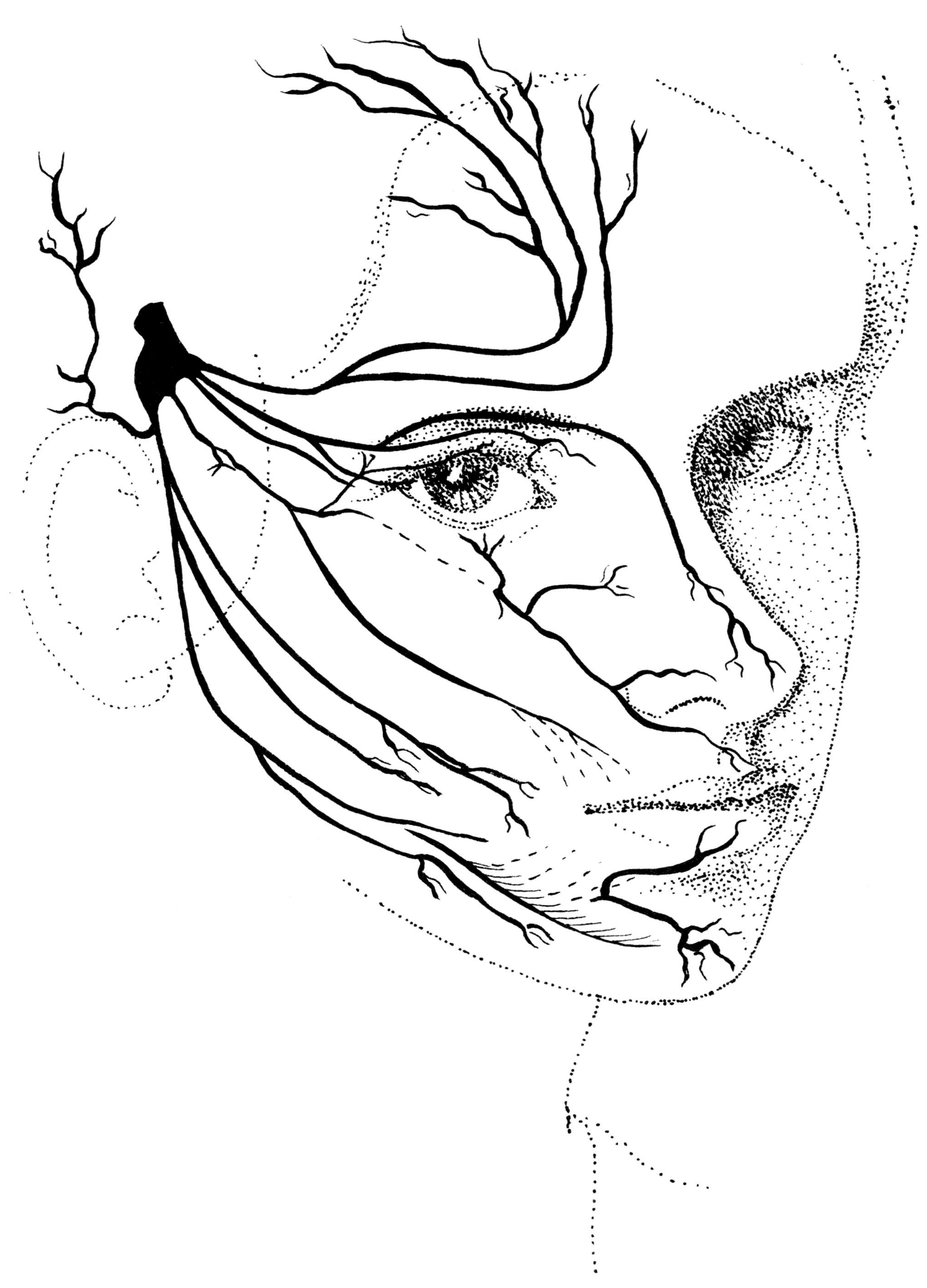

8. Head and Face

EXERCISE II

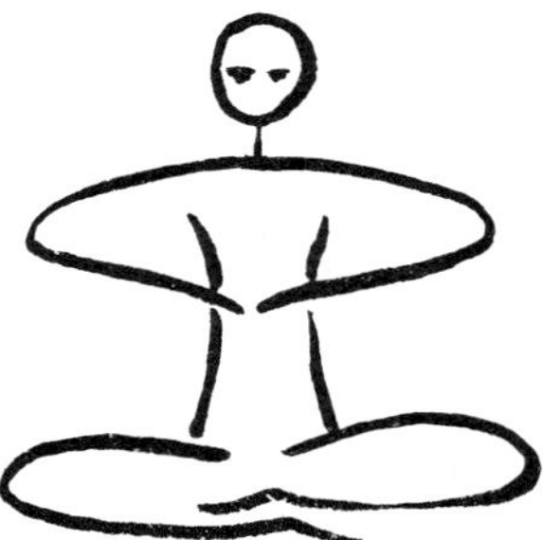

1. Sit in easy position. Raise elbows in horizontal position, hands hanging loosely in front of chest.

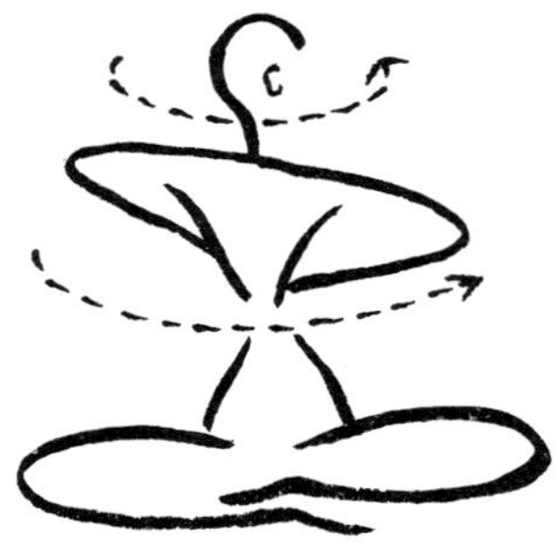

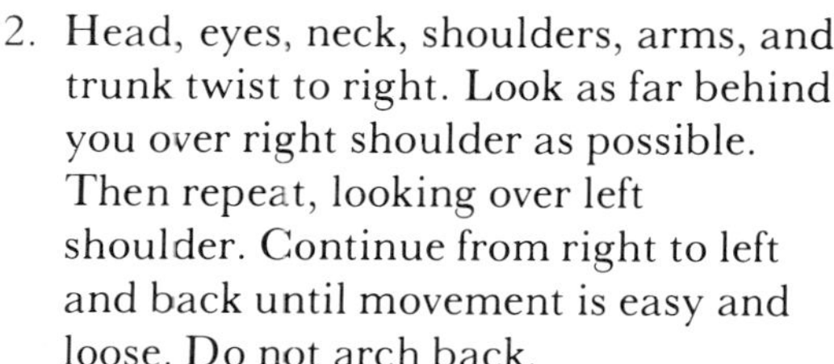

2. Head, eyes, neck, shoulders, arms, and trunk twist to right. Look as far behind you over right shoulder as possible. Then repeat, looking over left shoulder. Continue from right to left and back until movement is easy and loose. Do not arch back.

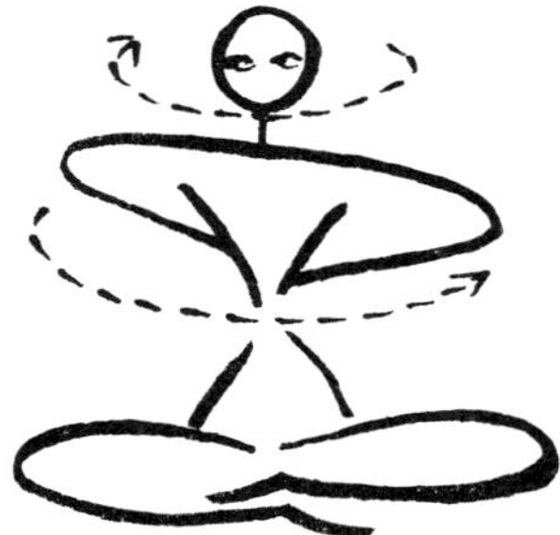

3. Move arms and shoulders to the right, head and eyes to the left. Repeat many times.

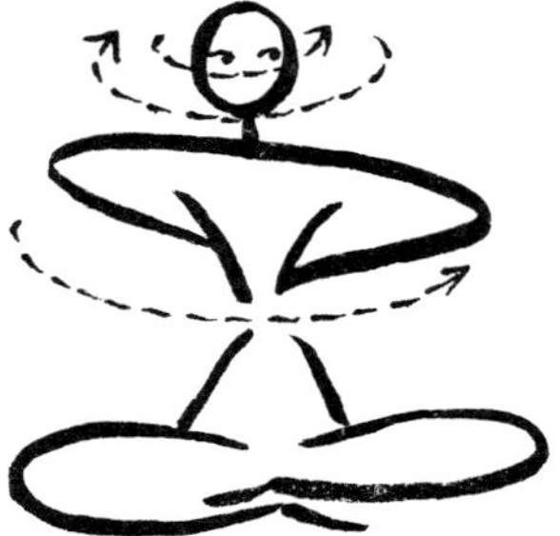

4. Now move arms and shoulders to the right, head to the left, and eyes to the right, as if following hands. Repeat many times, moving from side to side until action is easy.

EXERCISE III

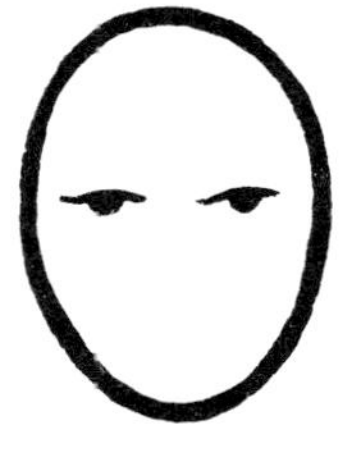

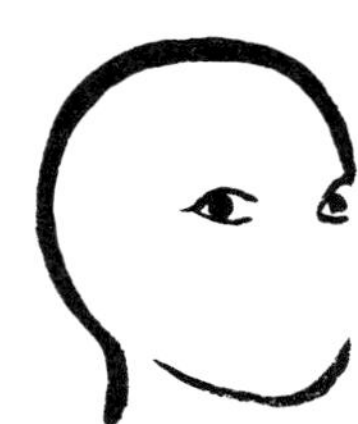

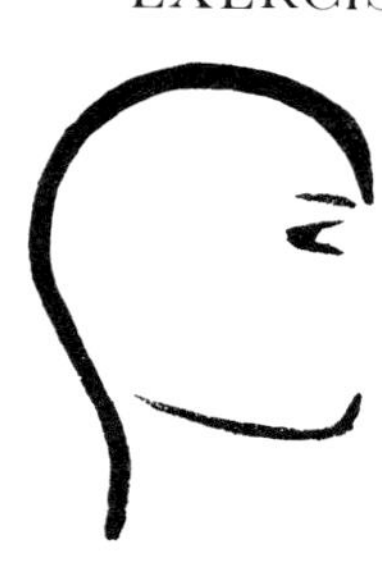

Focus eyes on a point in front of you. Turn head slowly to the left, while keeping eyes fixed on same point. Then turn head to the right. Repeat many times.

8. Head and Face

EXERCISE IV

This and other eye exercises will alter your perception of and place in the spatial world around you. With time, as your awareness improves, you will see and feel real changes in your body patterns.

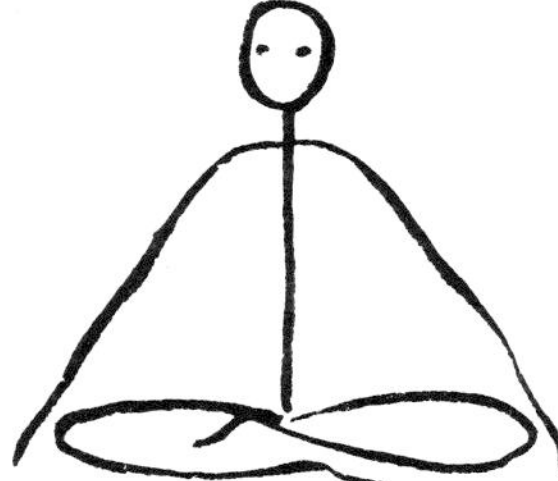

1. Sit in the easy position, wrists on knees. Neck, shoulders, arms, and hands relaxed. Eyes open.

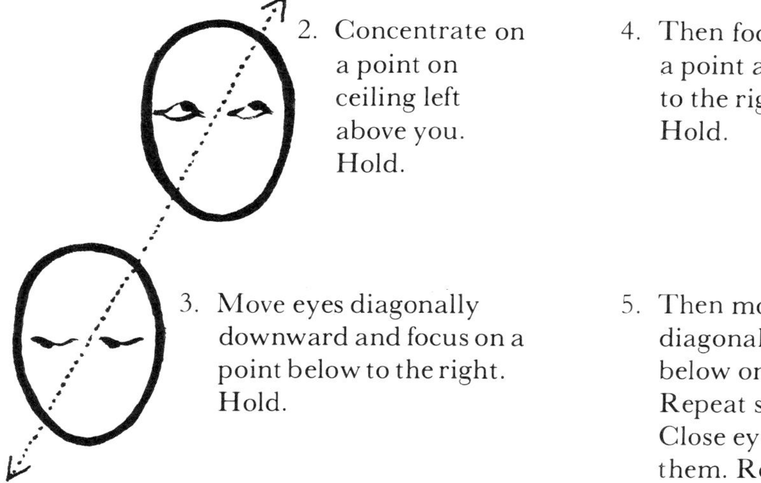

2. Concentrate on a point on ceiling left above you. Hold.

3. Move eyes diagonally downward and focus on a point below to the right. Hold.

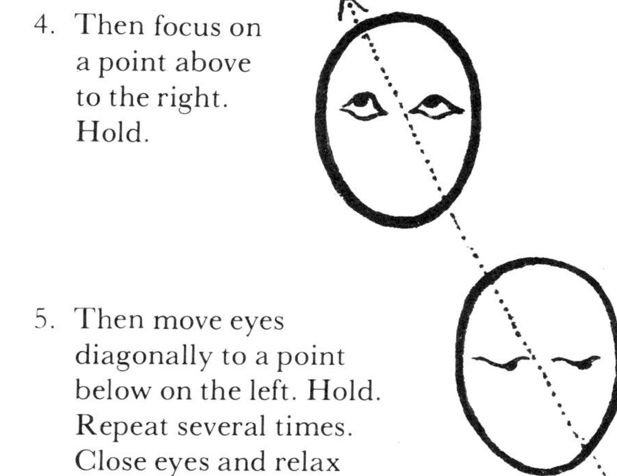

4. Then focus on a point above to the right. Hold.

5. Then move eyes diagonally to a point below on the left. Hold. Repeat several times. Close eyes and relax them. Relax rest of body.

EXERCISE V

Open your eyes. Look as far as possible in directions indicated below. Hold each gaze as long as comfortable, trying to focus on a specific point. Do not move the head.

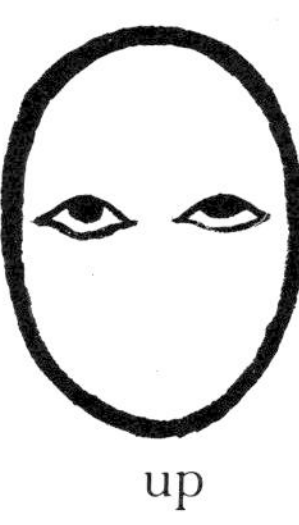

up

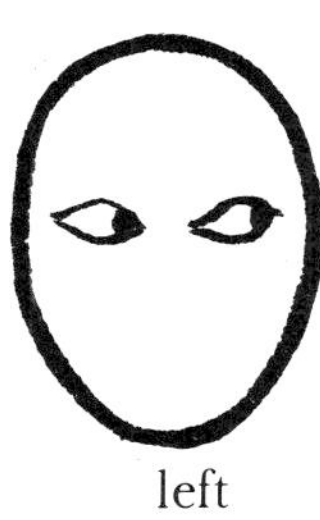

left

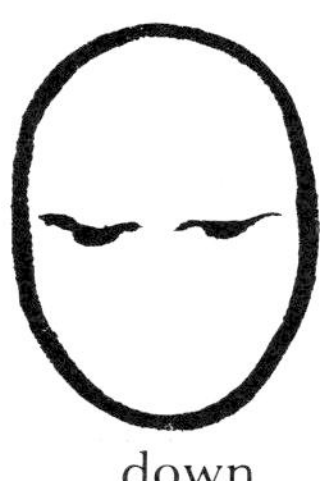

down

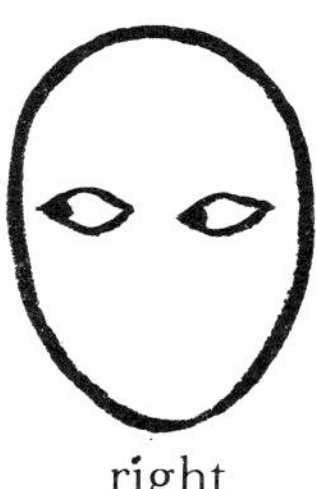

right

Then close your eyes and relax them. Check that your neck, shoulders, arms, and hands are relaxed.

EXERCISE VI

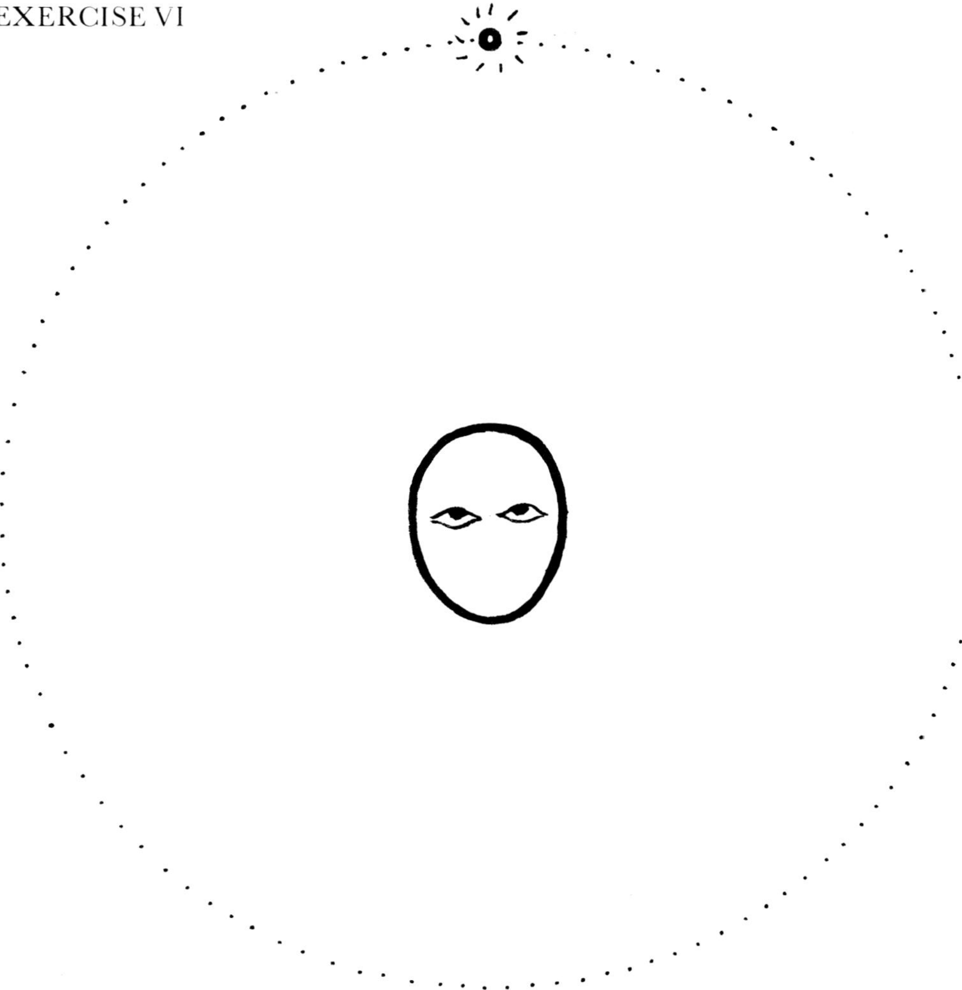

Open your eyes. Slowly move eyes in a circular movement around the room, making the circumference as wide as possible. Do not move head. Turn clockwise and anti-clockwise. Close your eyes and relax them.

EXERCISE VII

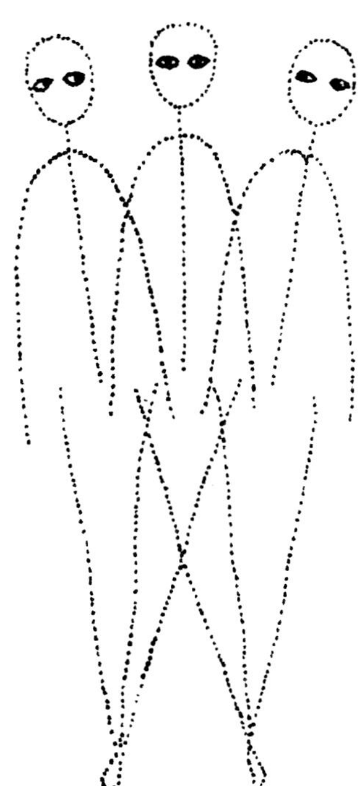

Stand with feet one foot apart. Focus eyes on a point across room. Keeping eyes fixed on same point, sway from side to side. Repeat many times.

EXERCISE VIII

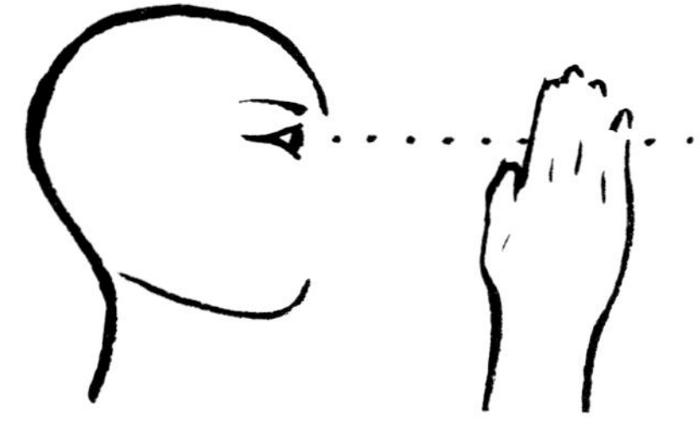

Sit in front of a window. Hold your hand one foot away from eyes. Focus eyes on hand. Then focus on a point outside the window as far away as possible. Then focus on hand again. Repeat many times.

EXERCISE IX

1. Lie down with eyes closed. Relax. Look in the black space in front of you. Among the flashes and sparkles that you may see, try to single out one dot and place it in front of you.

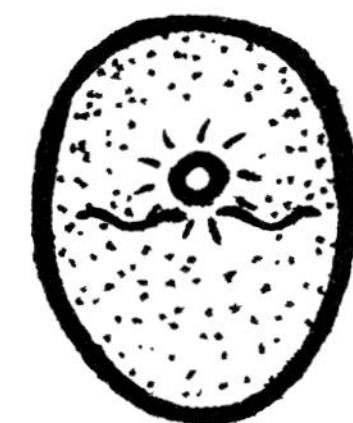

2. If you cannot fix the dot at one point, start by focusing your eyes in the centre of the space in front of you.

3. Imagine a horizon entering your field of vision in the East and leaving it in the West. Keep concentrating on the dot. Move dot over horizon from East to West and back again many times. If you cannot focus on a dot, move eyes over horizon. Move dot very slowly, like an airplane high in the sky, without jerks or jumps. Repeat many times until dot moves steadily. Hold it still at various intervals; then move it along again. Then place dot in centre of the horizon and move it from centre to right and back to centre many times. Then move dot from centre to left and back many times. Finally move dot from right to left and back again.

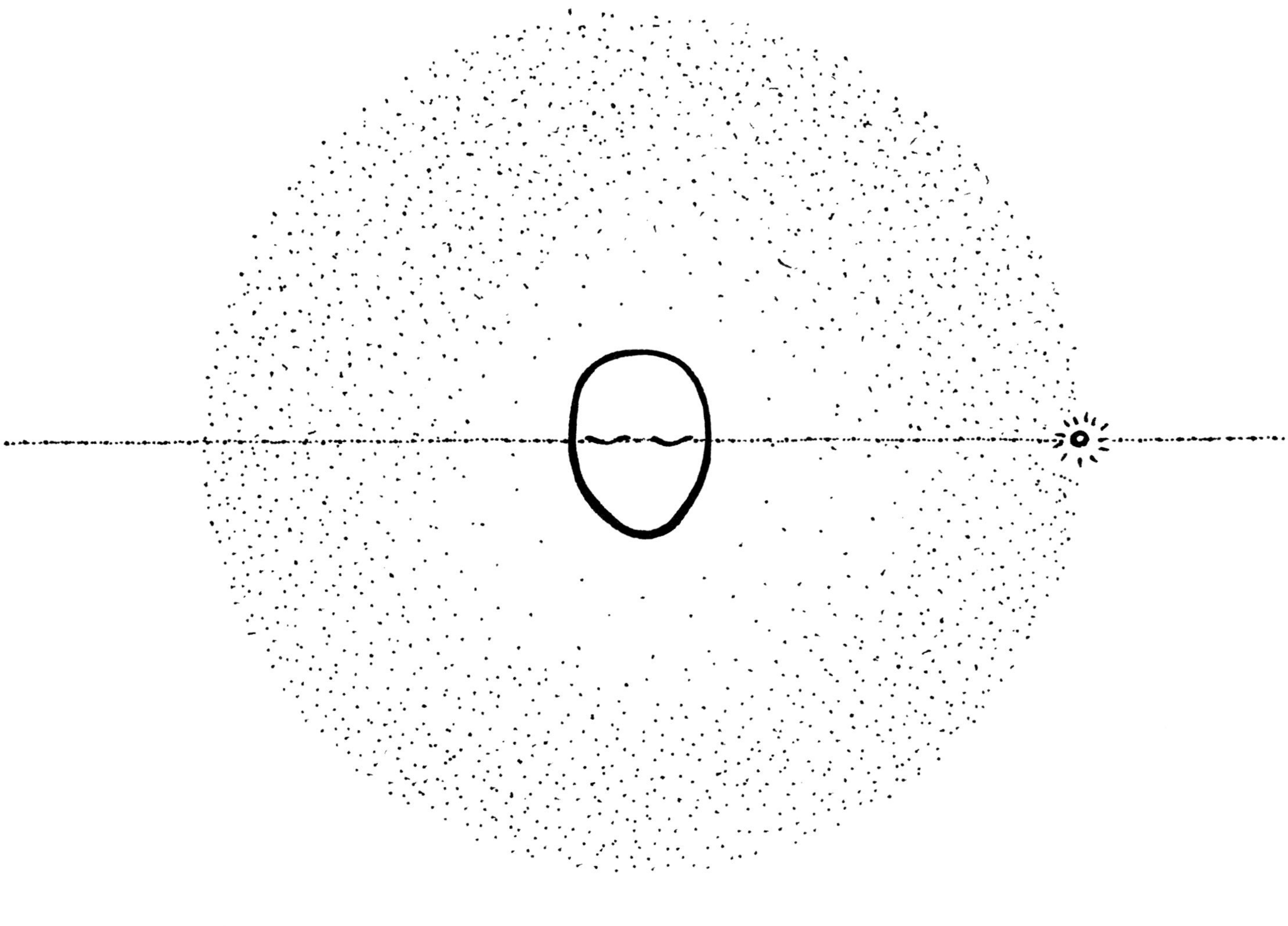

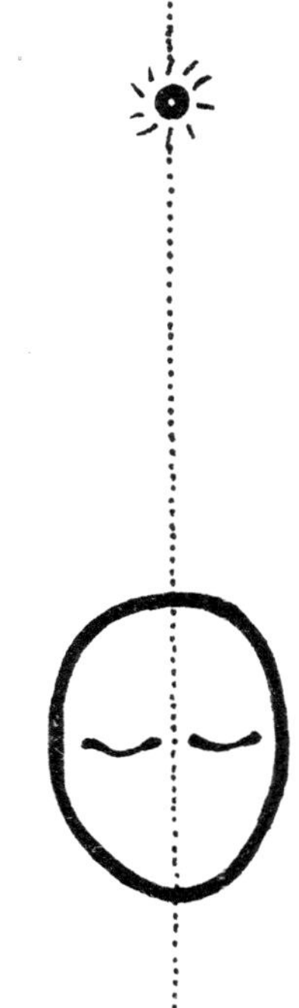

EXERCISE X

1. Imagine an arch over the body, from beyond the feet to over the head. Repeat movements from p. 103 vertically rather than horizontally. Observe which of two directions is easier for you. When the dot reaches the point where the arch touches the floor beyond your head, move eyes as if they are following the extension of the arch underneath your body. In the drawing below, the heavy black dots represent the first part of this exercise with arch over body, while the white dots represent continuation of arch below body.

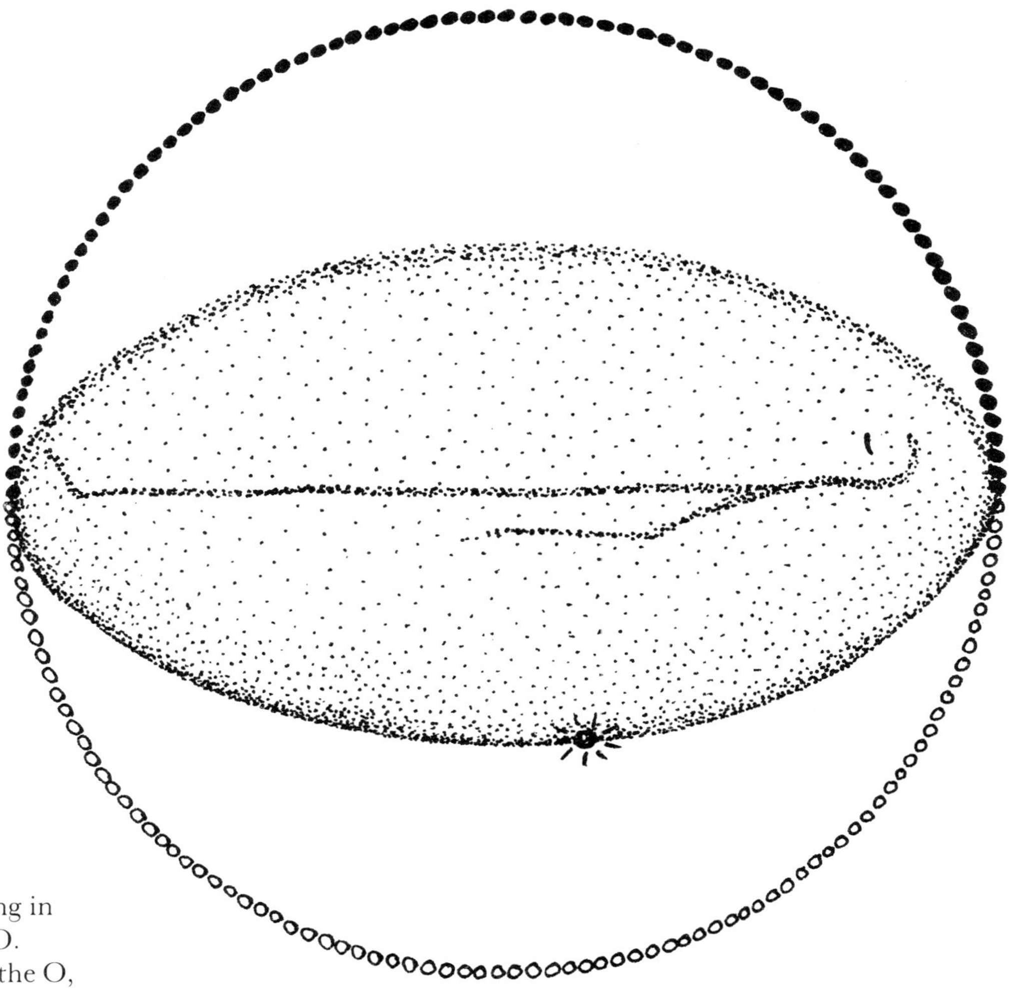

2. Now imagine you are lying in the centre of a big letter O. Slowly move dot around the O, as shown in drawing, clockwise and anti-clockwise. Relax.

EXERCISE XI

1. Still keeping eyes closed, imagine a big O in front of you. Place dot on top of O. Make dot travel slowly clockwise and anti-clockwise. Then relax eyes. Without touching eyes, cover them with hands.

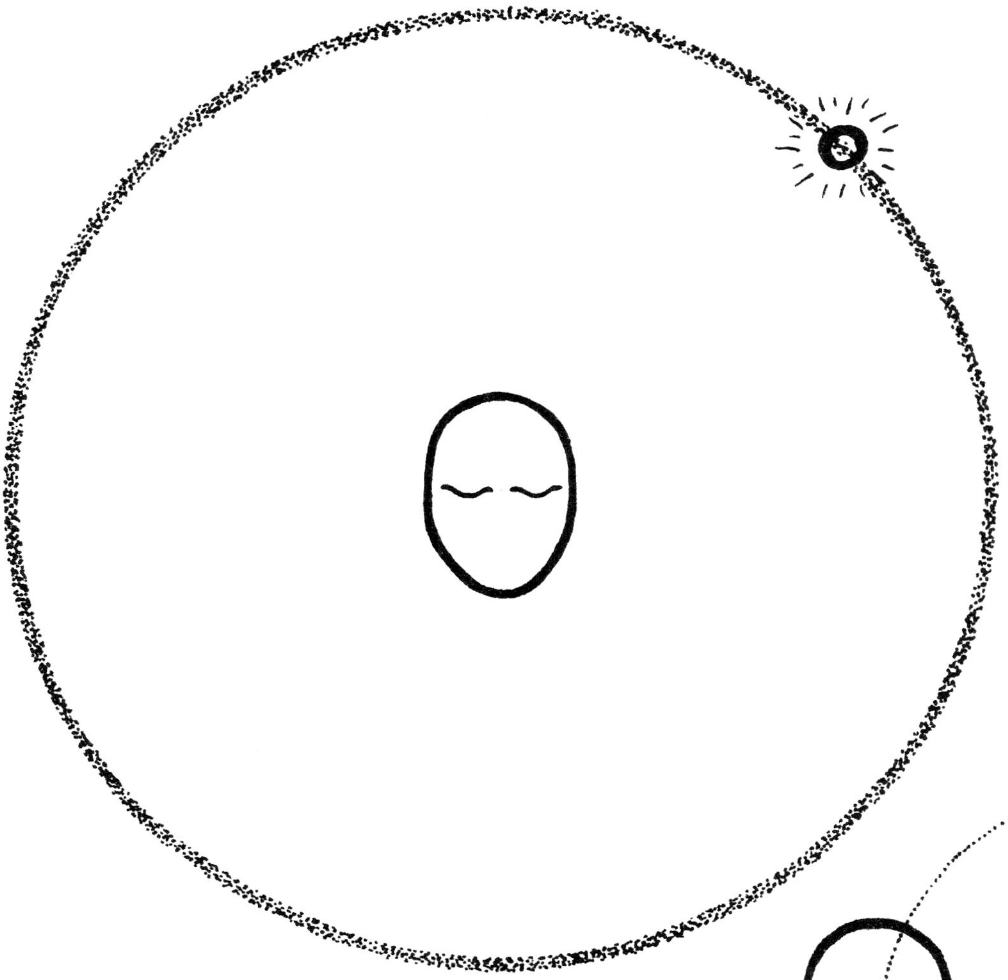

2. Concentrate on left eye. Imagine a circle in field of left eye only. Place dot on top of circle. Slowly follow dot around circle, clockwise and anti-clockwise. Relax. Repeat with right eye. Relax.

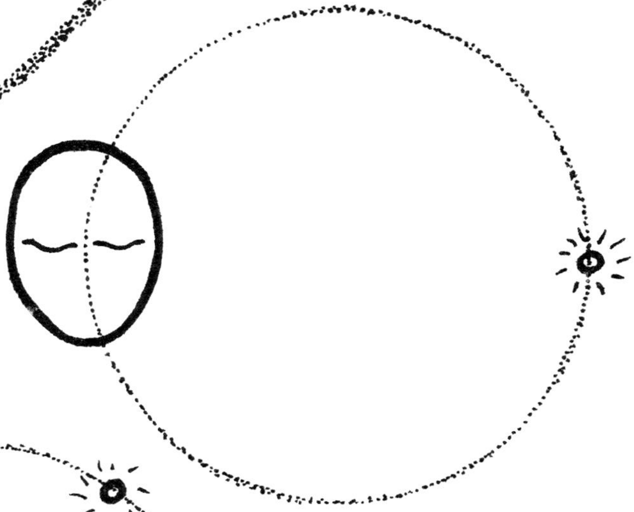

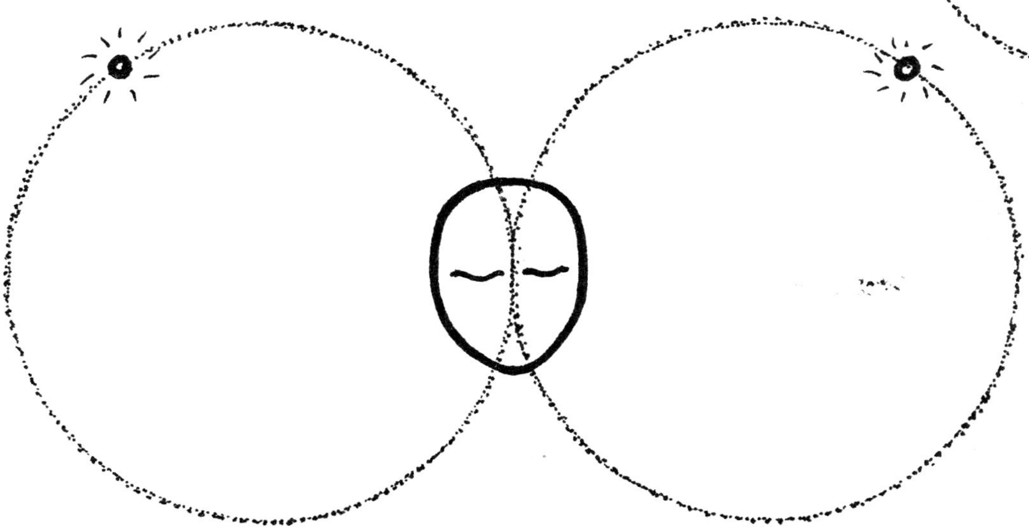

3. Now imagine two circles, one in field of right eye, one in field of left eye. Imagine you are going to sleep. Eyes roll back and outward. Place a dot on top of each circle. Move dots simultaneously in opposite directions until control comes. Then reverse directions of dots. Cover eyes to exclude all light. Relax.

EXERCISE XII

1. Imagine a feather floating from the ceiling straight down and landing on your forehead. between the eyebrows. Make it float up and down from forehead to ceiling many times.

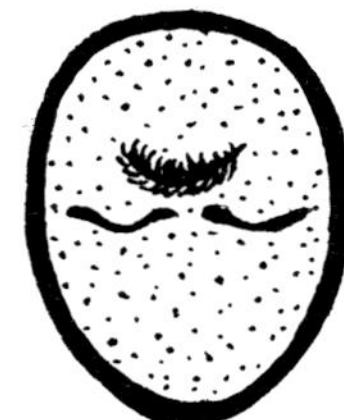

2. Stop feather between forehead and ceiling. Hold and move it at intervals. Relax. After practice you will find feather or dot moving itself. You must only follow it.

EXERCISE XIII

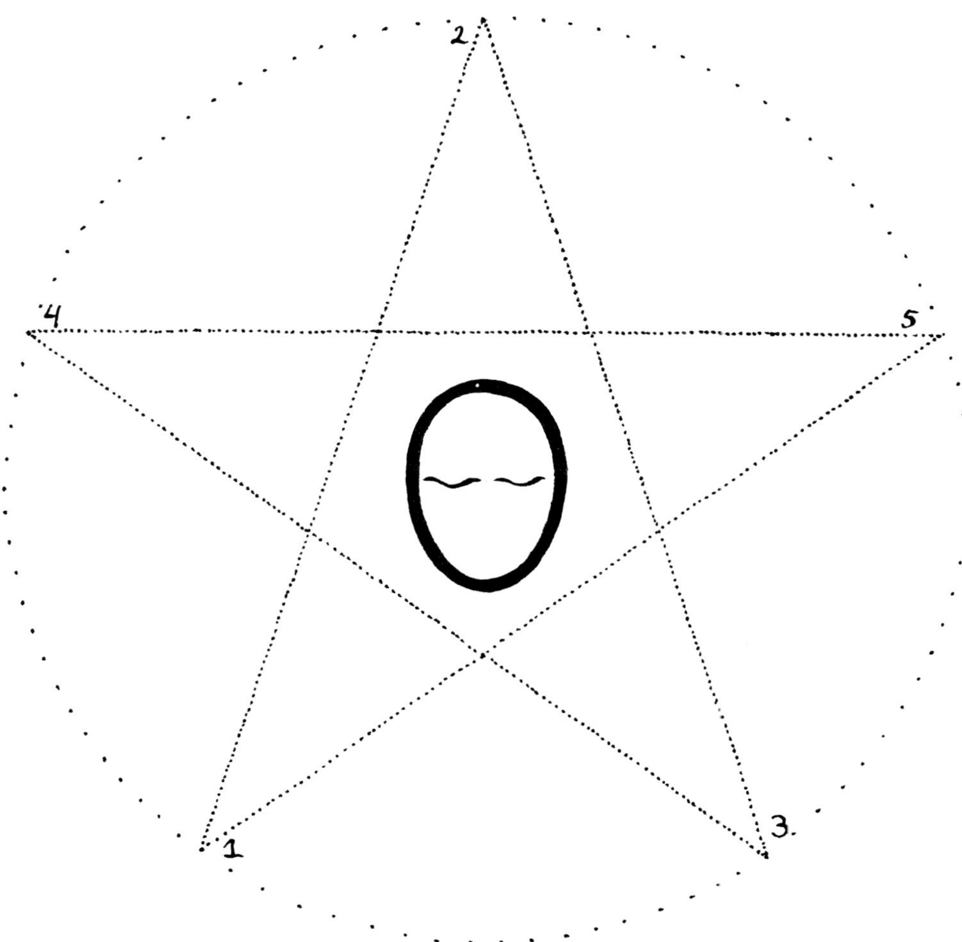

For this exercise imagine and draw a five-pointed star. Move dot to point 1; then to points 2, 3, 4, and 5. Return to starting point. Repeat several times, moving dot slowly and rhythmically. Relax eyes. Cup hands over eyes without touching them.

The mind's eye can also draw a triangle, square, number 8, and spiral.

9. PARTNER YOGA

Although this book is entitled *Feel Yourself*, the title does not imply that feeling another is wrong or superfluous. Feeling yourself is only a beginning. In many cases exercising with someone else is extremely practical, as it may be initially difficult for you to maintain a suggested contact with the floor. A partner can help by exerting a small amount of pressure on your legs or shoulders or back to stretch and loosen desired areas. It is certainly emotionally satisfying to share with a friend or loved one the growing awareness of your body's potentiality. This increasing sensitivity and strength can be directed towards another with beneficial and often wonderful results.

Now that you have spent some time working from foot to head of your own body, several exercises are listed which call more explicitly for two people. You may wish to precede these efforts with some of your favourite loosening-up exercises. The energy from within each of you will flow out and be returned.

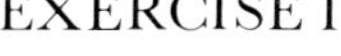

EXERCISE I

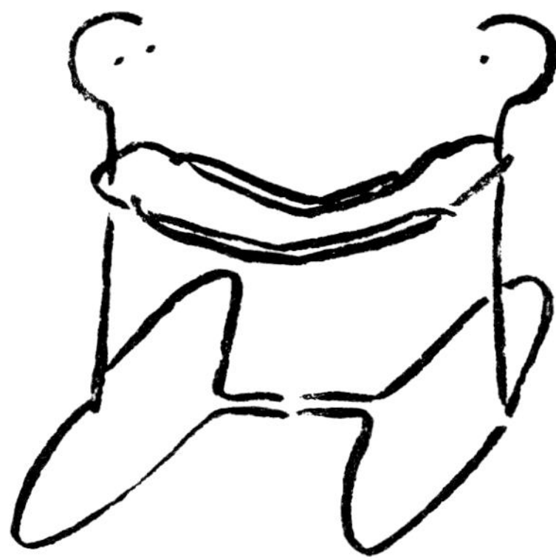

1. Sit in tailor position on floor in front of each other, toes touching. Hold Carol's hands or elbows.

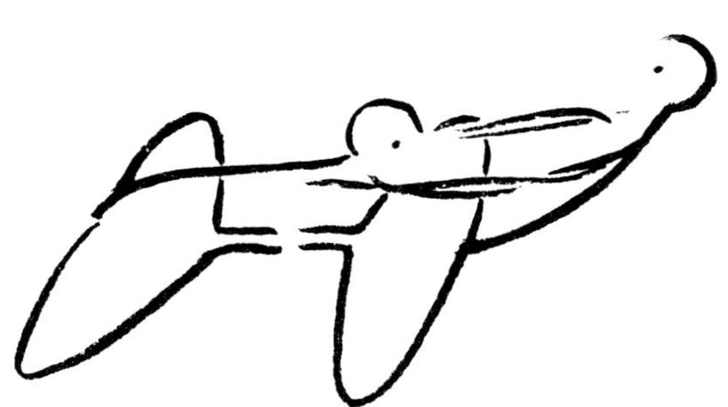

2. Lean backward while pulling Carol forward. You both should keep buttocks on floor. Hold as long as pleasant.

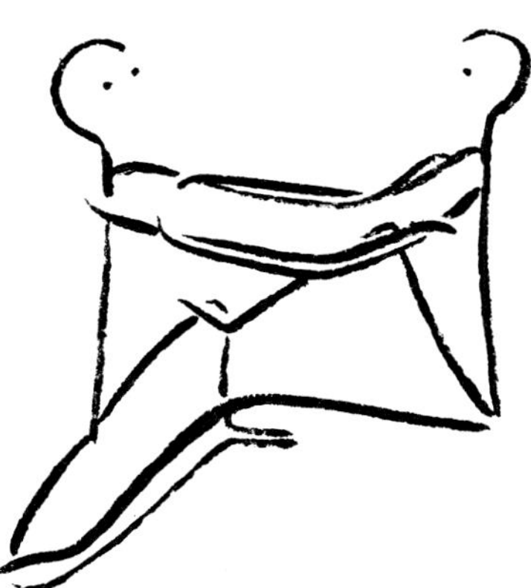

3. Place your feet on her knees, gently pressing them downward.

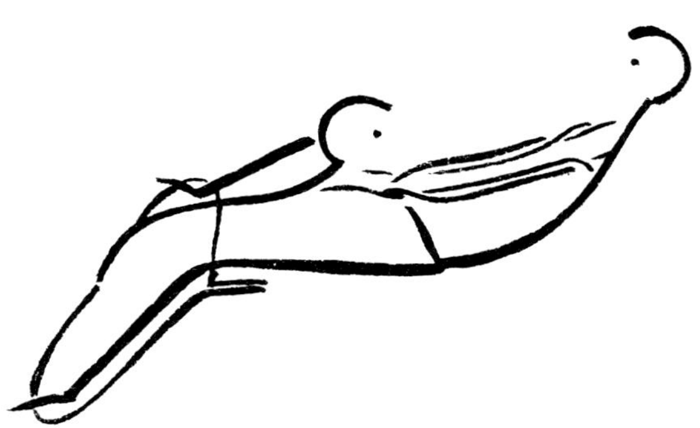

4. Lean backward and pull Carol forward. Hold as long as possible. Let her pull you forward.

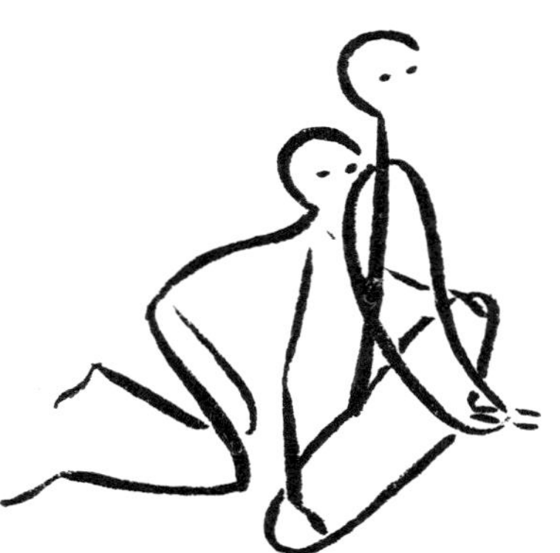

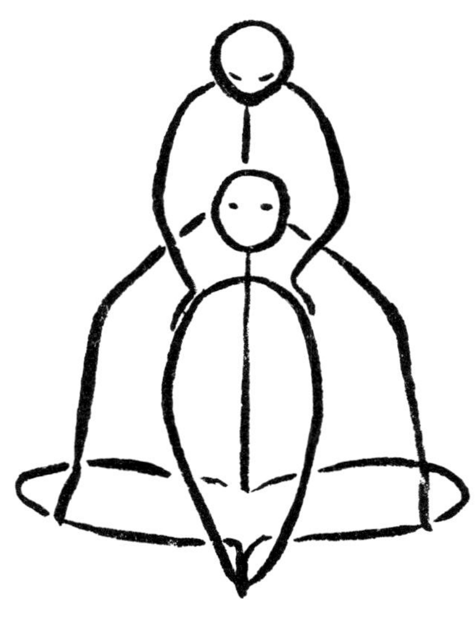

EXERCISE II

1. Marius sits in tailor position; stand or kneel behind him. With both hands push his knees toward floor.

2. If Marius is still happy with the feeling, place your feet on his knees, rest your hands on his shoulders, and then stand on his knees. Try not to go past limits of what feels good.

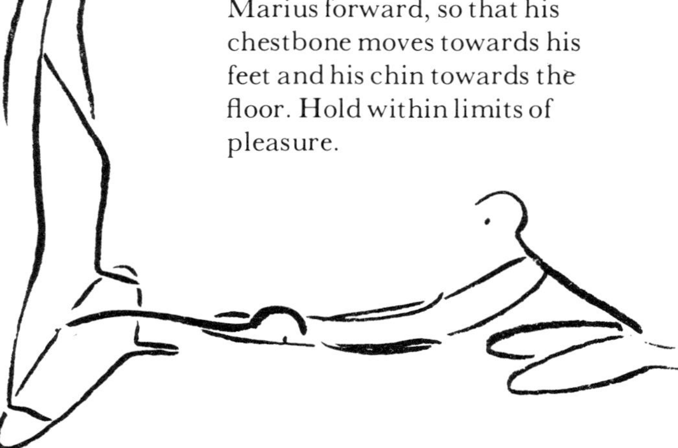

3. Still standing on Marius' knees, ask Diana to pull Marius forward, so that his chestbone moves towards his feet and his chin towards the floor. Hold within limits of pleasure.

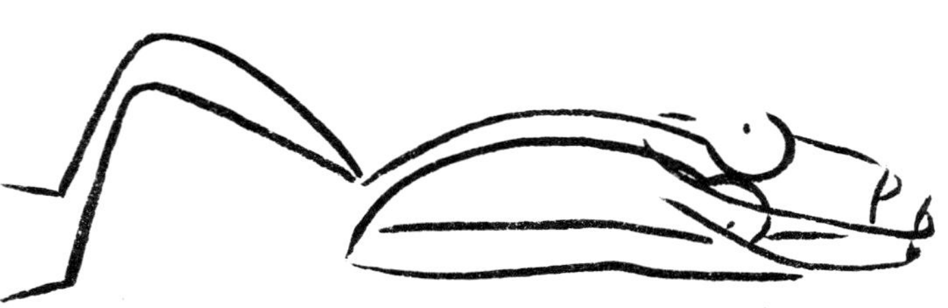

EXERCISE III

Christen and you sit back to back, her legs straight and feet together. Christen takes hold of her feet (or back of knees, calves, or ankles). Place your tailbone against her lower back and lie back on it. Back of your skull should touch back of her skull. Then stretch arms over your head and try to take hold of Christen's feet. Both of you should relax. By gently rocking from right to left and rubbing your spine forward and backward over Christen's spine, her back will relax more and more until she sinks down further and further. Hold as long as enjoyable.

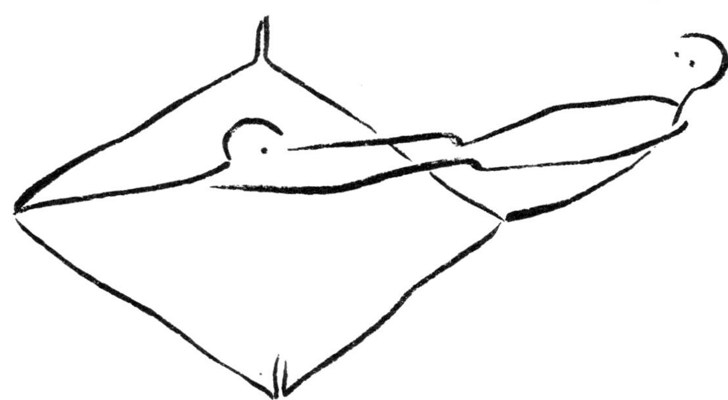

EXERCISE IV

Sit on floor facing each other. Spread legs as wide apart as possible. Press bottoms of feet together. Hold Sid's hands or elbows. Slowly lean backward while pulling Sid forward. Continue as long as it is pleasant for him. Repeat several times. Then let Sid pull you forward.

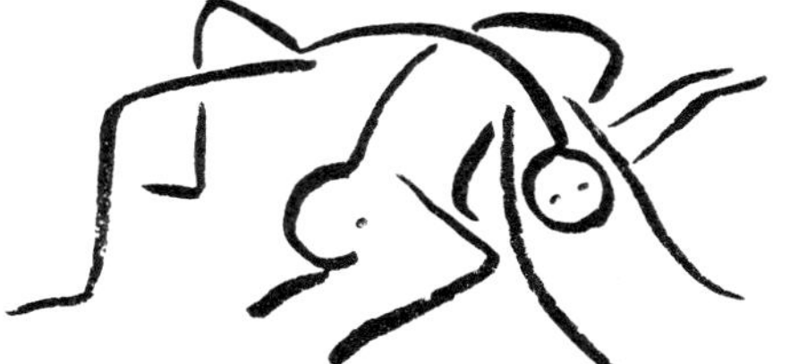

EXERCISE V

1. Kneel down with elbows on floor. Joy stands next to you and lies down backward over you. Her feet on one side, head and arms hang over other side.

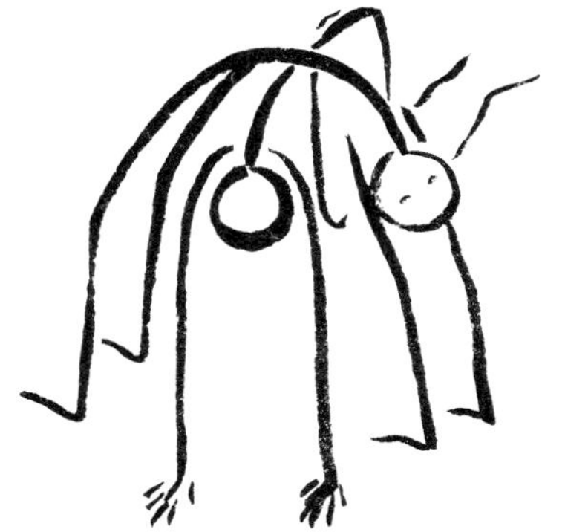

2. Depending on Joy's looseness, straighten arms and raise her upward, increasing arch of spine – but watch that you don't tip her off. Joy's hands and feet may leave floor. All she needs do is relax. When Joy has stretched enough in this position, sink down and let her slide off your back. Reverse positions.
   Try another way of getting into this stretch. Carol gets in backward bend. Then crawl under her back and push your back upward, increasing her backward bend. Hold within limits of pleasure. Then by pushing your back still further up, help Carol to come up standing from the bend.

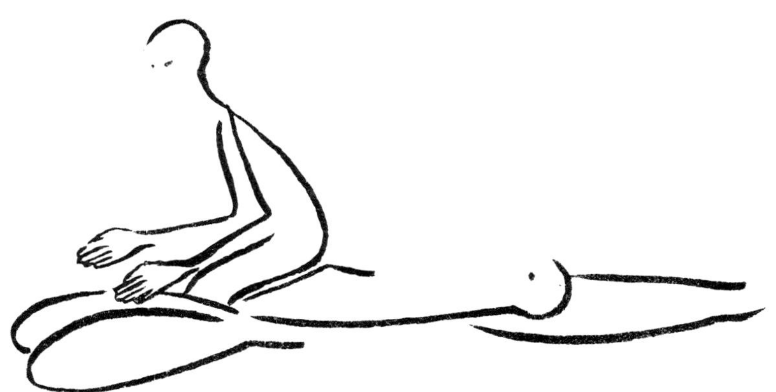

EXERCISE VI

Lie on back, arms over head, knees bent, feet curled round buttocks. If this is too difficult, bend one leg and keep other straight. What Bill can do: Rub and stroke thighs to relieve tension in stretched muscles. Then strike thighs as follows: hands loosely together, palms inward. With wrists relaxed, outside of left hand hits thigh with gentle blow, immediately followed by similar tap of right hand. Continue as long as comfortable.

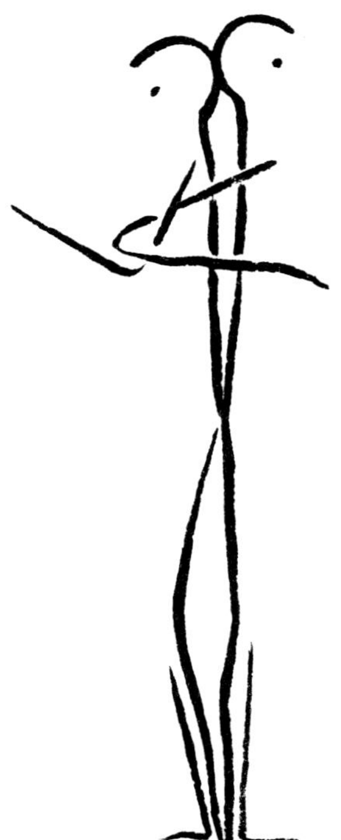

EXERCISE VII

1. Stand back to back. Hook your arms in Miriam's arms and hold them in firm lock.

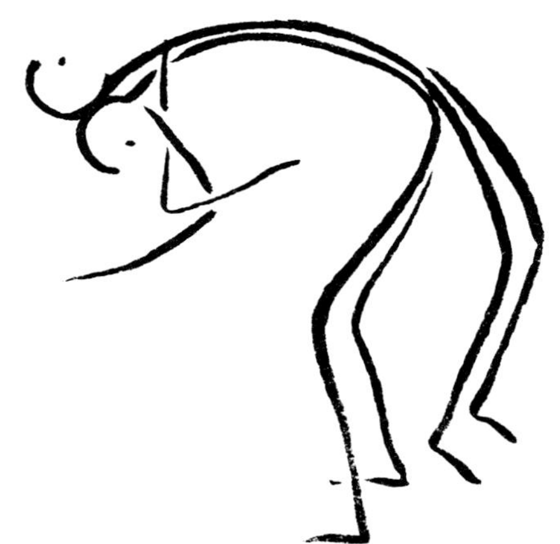

2. Bend knees slightly, placing your tailbone under Miriam's tailbone. Bend forward while she leans backward. Her spine rests on yours, her feet come off floor. It is possible to support people bigger than you. Miriam should relax her body totally. Round your spine and gently move from side to side or up and down, whatever feels good. Come up and let her feet touch floor. Then Miriam bends forward and you lie back, spine upon spine.

EXERCISE VIII

Niva assumes position as shown in second drawing on p. 49. With gentle rotating movements Yael massages pressure points in Niva's lower back on either side of spine, starting with tailbone and slowly moving up, vertebra by vertebra, careful not to push down. Yael also massages buttocks in area around hip joints. Yael holds Niva's feet together and on floor. Niva's pelvis will sink downward as Yael's massage relieves any tension. Carry on as long as pleasant for both of you. Then reverse positions.

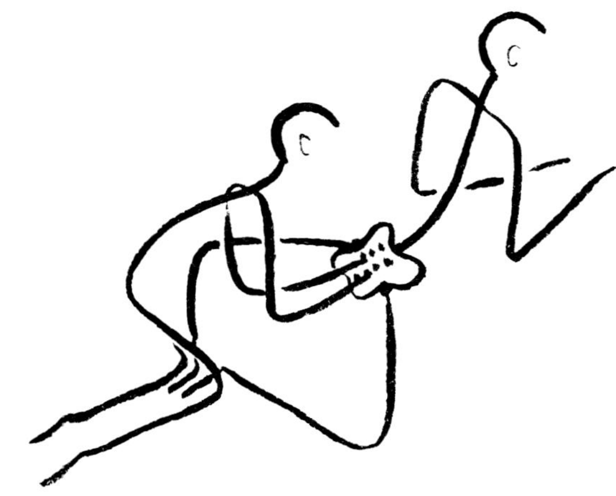

EXERCISE IX

Kelly and Tasnima stand two arm lengths away from each other, holding hands, arms straight. Keeping heels on floor, they float down to a squatting position and rise again together.

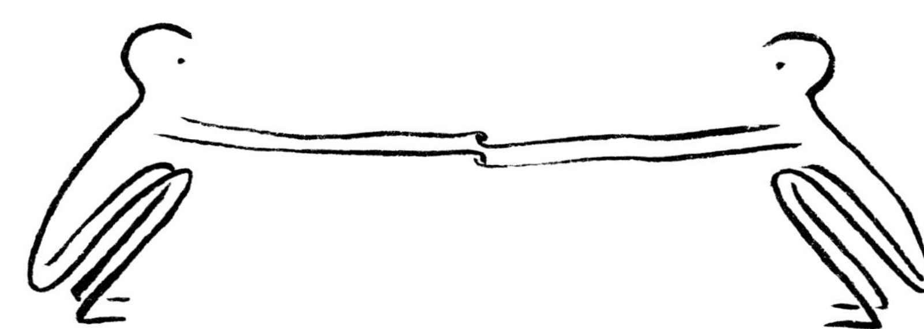

10. BALANCE

Watching trapeze artists performing at a circus, we are amazed by their grace and balance. Watch an animal run, climb, hunt, or chase another animal. Action is instinctive; movement and balance are one. Yet, most of us feel terribly earthbound and gravity-controlled as we move about in our daily life, spending most of our time in standing, sitting, or prone positions. Simply thinking about the people on the flying trapeze is dizzying. How can they maintain their sense of balance?

The sense of balance depends upon input from the eyes (in response to head movement); nerve endings in muscles, tendons, and joints; pressure-sensitive points in the soles of the feet; and the complex organs of the inner ear. The labyrinth of the inner ear is the equilibrium centre. It contains two fluid sacs and three semi-circular canals, each at right angles to the other two. Shifting body and head affects the level of fluid in the canals. We are accustomed to movements in the horizontal plane, both left-right and forward-backward (as when walking). Movement in the vertical plane (as in an elevator) can produce dizziness and a feeling of loss of equilibrium. In this chapter the head will find itself in many extraordinary places. We shall try to become as much at ease on one foot as two, with head below shoulders as well as above. At one point your body balanced quite naturally with head and shoulders below. For most of us our head and shoulders were first to appear in the outside world. We must re-learn what was previously natural.

Balance is a mental as well as a physical state. Some of the exercises in this chapter may make you feel clumsy and awkward at first. But proceed, while remembering that the necessary physical balance comes slowly and as a result of relaxation and stillness of mind. Tension and anxiety are not conducive to creating a sense of balance. The circle is completed when you experience the transitions from relaxation to physical balance to increased stillness of mind with heightened self-awareness. The eyes-closed exercises necessitate creation of a point of focus inside. In the turning exercises, outer reference points become unfixed and meaningful only in relation to the 'centre' point which is you and the balance you have created within you.

EXERCISE I

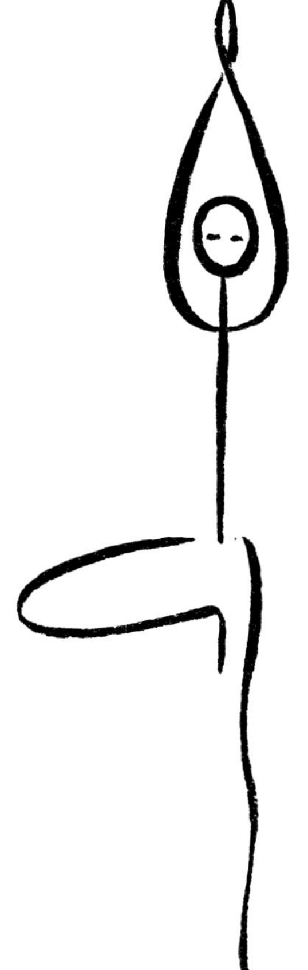

1. Stand with feet together, toes pointing forward. Place right foot on inside of left thigh. Stretch arms up and cross left wrist in front of right. Twist wrists and bring palms together. Arms straight, elbows behind ears. Eyes focus on a fixed points in front of you.
   Balance.
   Come back to standing position and repeat on other side.

2. Repeat previous exercise with right foot now as high as up in left groin as possible.

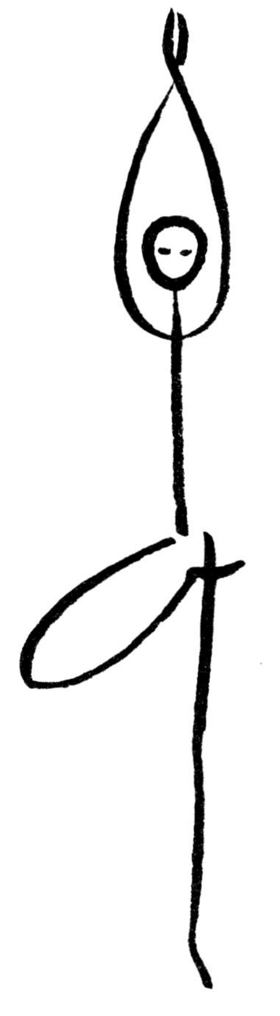

EXERCISE II

1. Stand with feet one foot apart, toes pointed forward, eyes closed. Slowly move body as if describing a circle on ceiling with top of head. Movement comes from ankles, easy and flowing. Move clockwise and anti-clockwise.

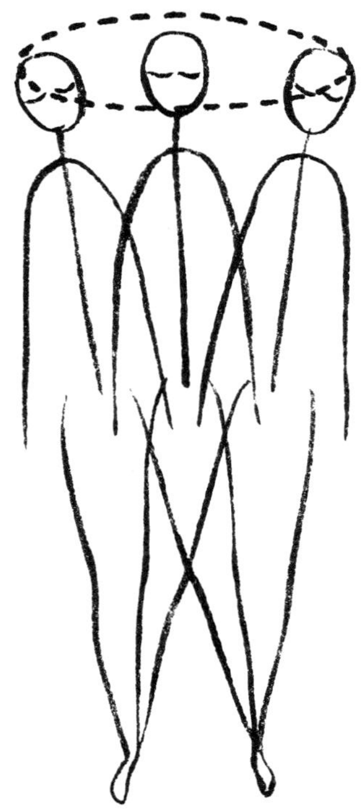

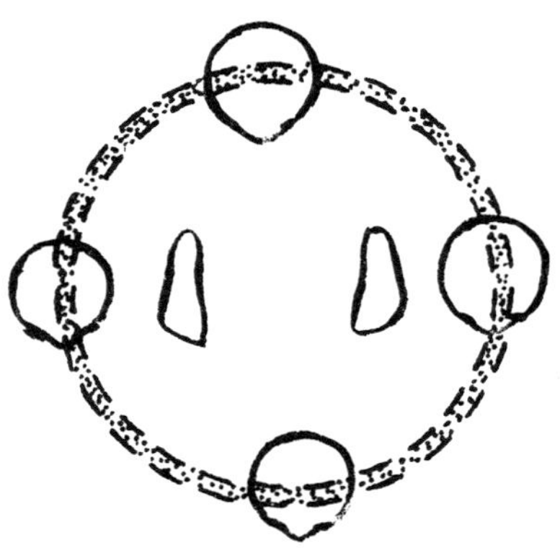

Seen from above.

2. Still keeping eyes closed, divide weight of body over both feet. Rock from right to left and back, keeping both feet firmly planted on floor. Rock many times. Gradually come to a standstill.

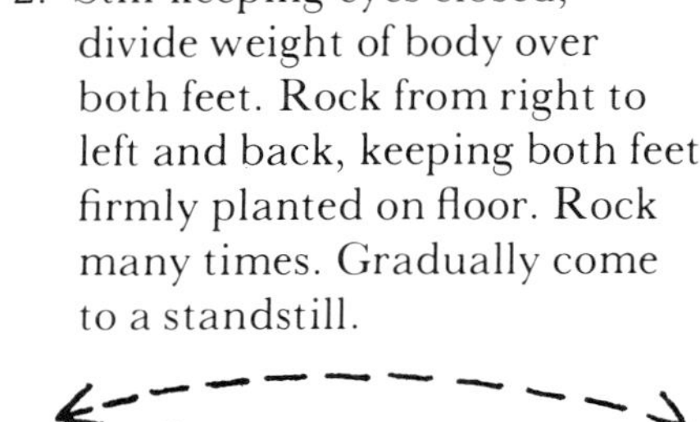

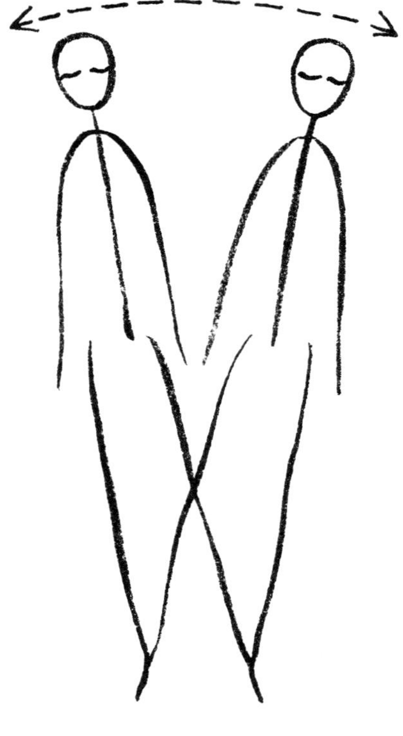

EXERCISE III

After these movement exercises, repeat either of the two balance exercises on p. 109 or the following: Feet together, toes forward, eyes closed. Bend right knee, moving right foot behind right thigh. Hold foot with right hand and pull it upward and backward. Stretch left arm up. Drop head back. Balance. Come back to standing position and repeat on other side.

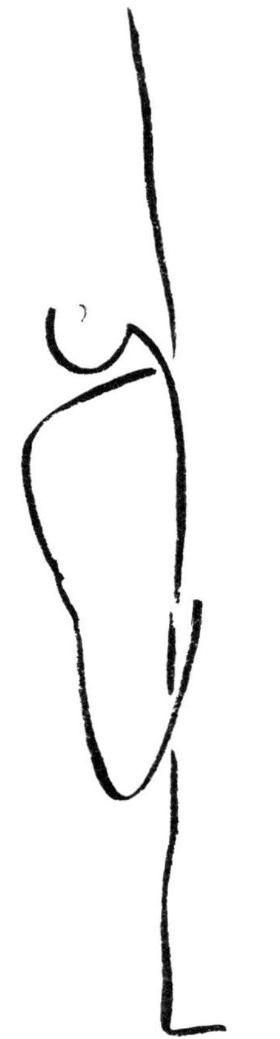

EXERCISE IV

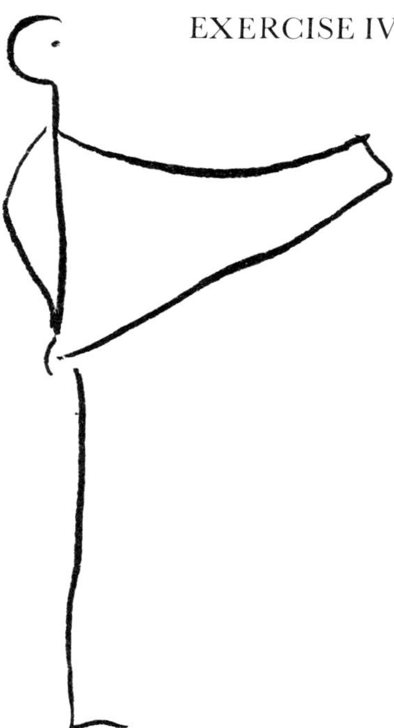

1. Stand with feet together, hands on hips. Pull right knee toward chest. Index and middle fingers of right hand hook big toe of right foot. Straighten right leg. Keep spine straight. Hold as long as comfortable. Repeat on left side.

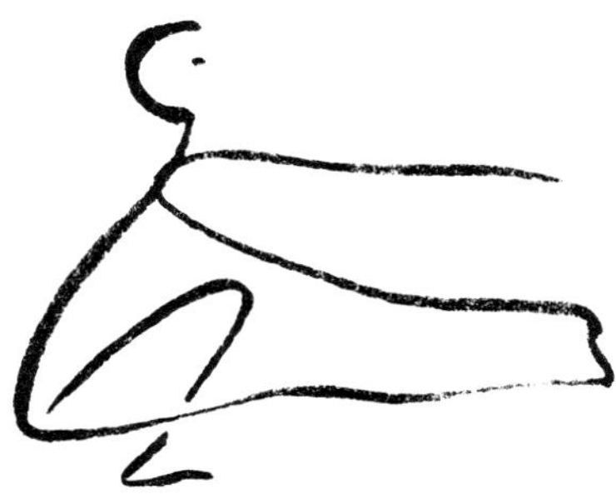

2. While in above position, stretch left arm forward. Bend left leg and slowly sink to squatting position on left foot, left heel on floor. Right leg stays off floor. Straighten left leg and slowly stand up. Repeat on other side.

EXERCISE V

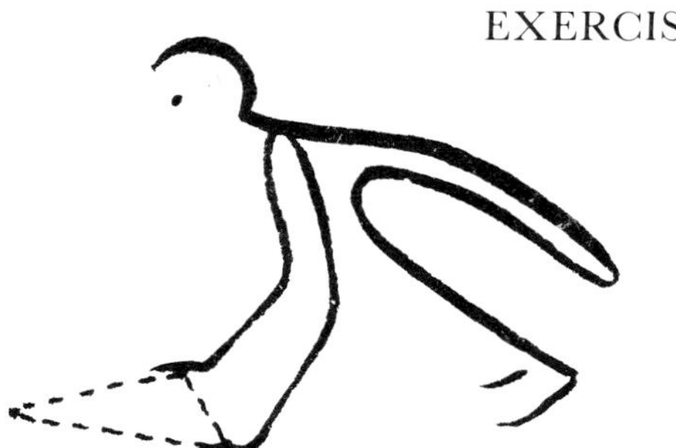

1. Crouch down. Hands on floor in front of you, in line with shoulders. Choose and concentrate on a point on floor as the top of a triangle with hands as base of triangle.

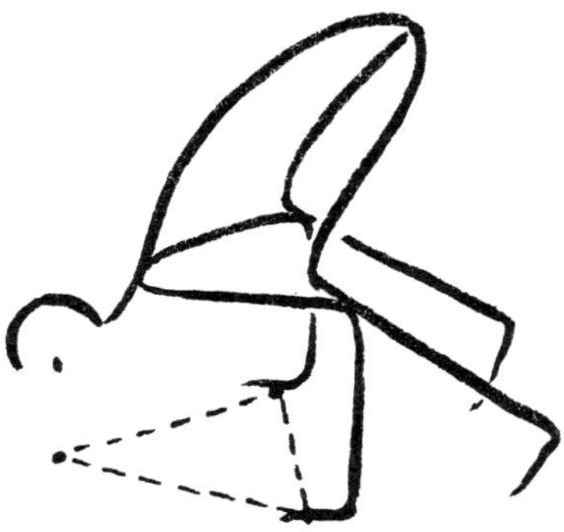

2. Raise hips and stand on toes. Move trunk forward. Upper arms and forearms perpendicular. Elbows stay above hands, shoulder width apart. Place knees on back of elbows. Eyes remain fixed on reference point.

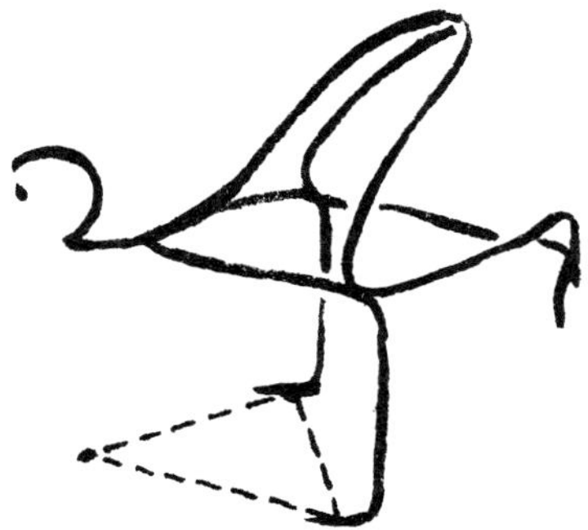

3. Transfer weight of body slowly on to elbows, until toes leave floor. Do not jump. Maintain balance. Cross ankles, arch spine, and look up. Reverse movements to return to crouching position.

EXERCISE VI: WHIRLING

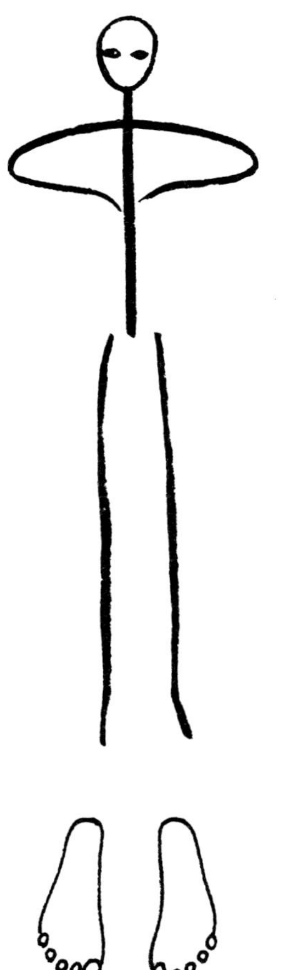

1. Whirling is not as complicated as it sounds. Maintain a three-beat cadence. To start, stand with feet slightly apart, toes forward. Raise elbows to the side, hands in front of you relaxed, palms down. Eyes focus on a reference point at eye level in front of you.

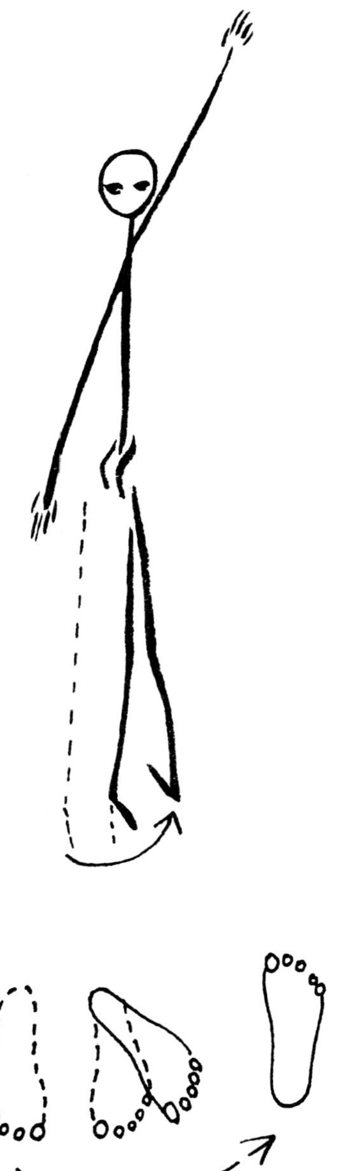

2. Right foot crosses over left foot and rests on floor about six inches away from left foot, with toes pointed toward wall behind you. At same time left foot makes a quarter turn. Spread arms horizontally, palms upward. As trunk makes a quarter turn with first step of left foot, right arm points towards reference point, left arm stretches toward wall behind you. Eyes remain fixed on original reference point.

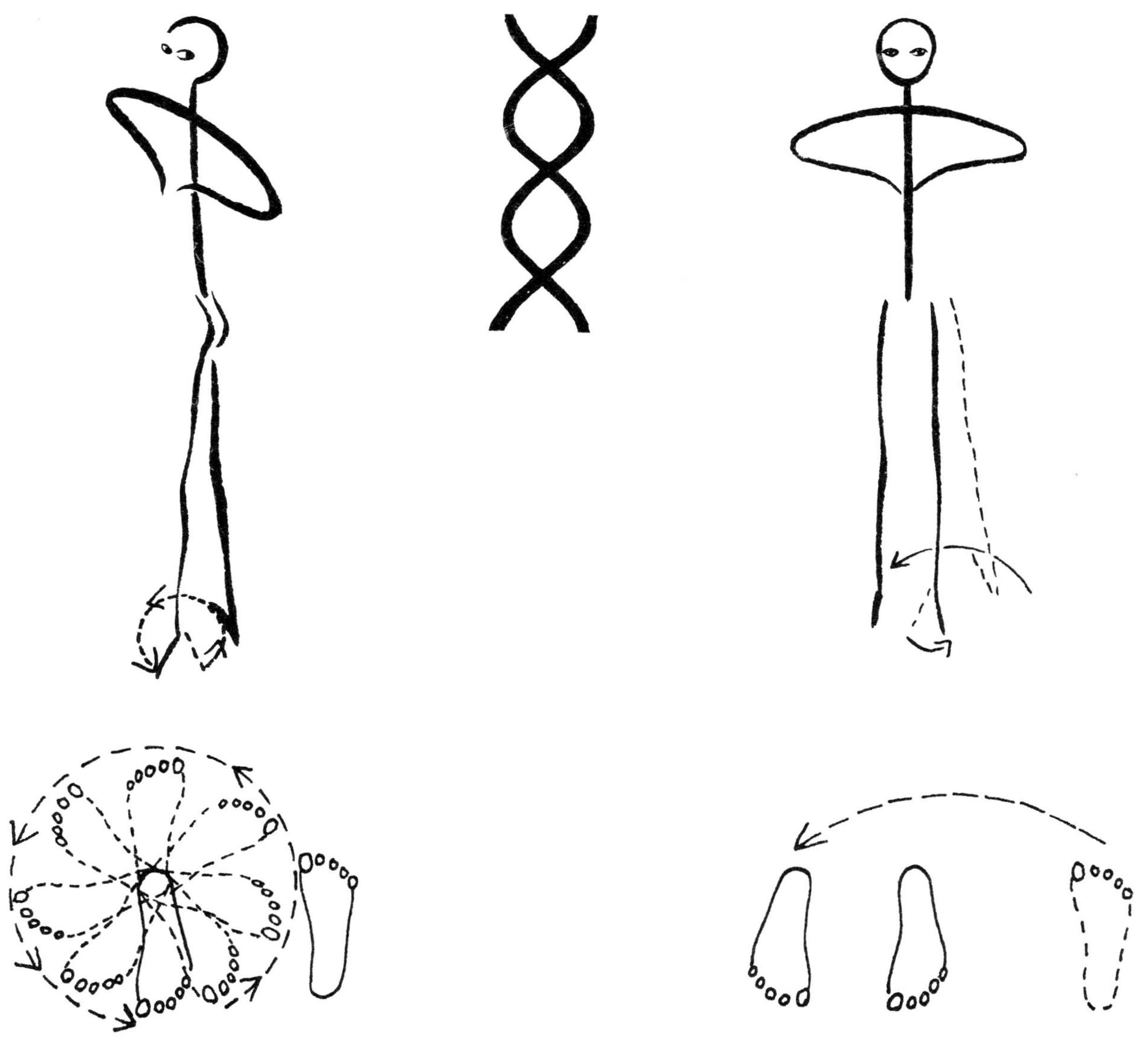

3. Keeping heel of left foot on floor, raise ball of left foot and turn it toward wall behind you. Continue turn right round, so that left foot returns to its starting position. Bring both hands in front of chest again. As body turns, eyes lose the reference point. Your gaze travels around room, sees wall behind you, and returns to reference point.

4. Then place right foot next to left foot again. Both feet are back in starting position, whole body faces forward, having turned round completely. Arms remain in same position, eyes fixed on original point. With practice, this turning will become smooth and fast. Try it turning in the opposite direction.

EXERCISE VII

The muscles that normally hold the body erect are constantly affected by gravity. In the headstand muscles are still relating to gravity, but in reverse fashion. This improves posture and enhances coordination and relaxation.

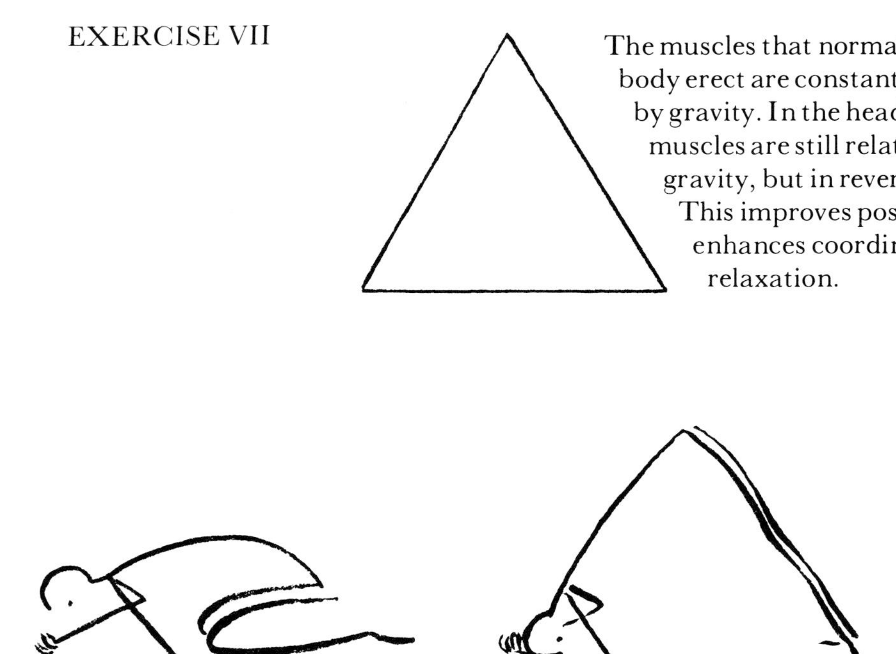

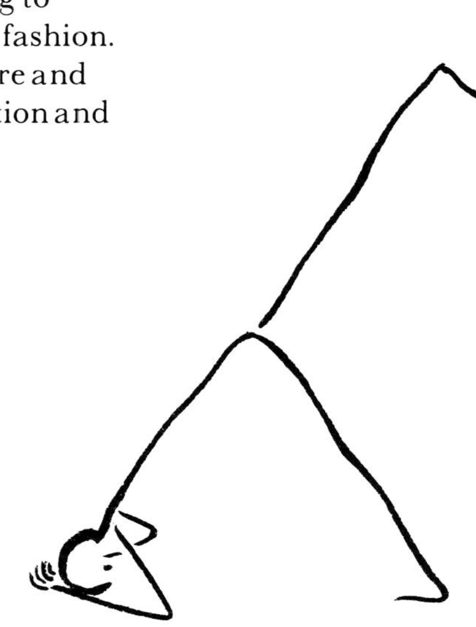

1. Place elbows on floor, straight under shoulders. Interlace fingers; thumbs cross over each other. Elbows form two lower points of a triangle, hands the top. Triangle gives stability to the posture.
2. Tuck toes under and straighten legs.
3. Raise right leg and stretch it upward. Dig left heel into floor. Straighten spine. Repeat with other leg. Return to position 2.

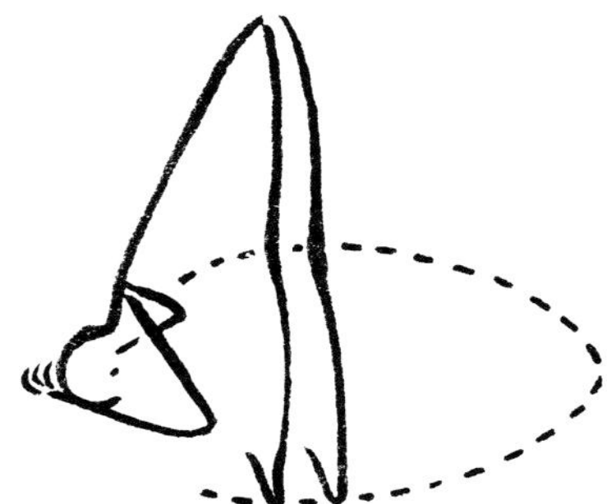

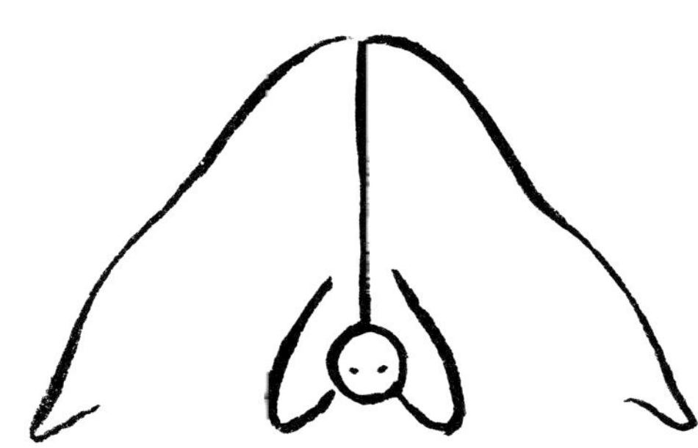

4. Without moving elbows, walk with small steps to the right. Keep feet as close in to head as possible. Hold. Walk back to starting point and continue on to the left.
5. Start in position 2. Walk both feet as close to head as possible. Then spread them as far apart as possible. Straighten legs. Push heels toward floor. Push armpits in direction of knees. Tuck tailbone upward and backward. Hold. Release and relax.

EXERCISE VIII: HEADSTAND

1. Place top of head on floor, so that back of head touches hands. Straighten legs; tuck toes under. Walk feet in direction of head. Straighten spine until back comes in vertical position. Pelvis moves upward and slightly backward, lifting legs off floor. Do not jump. Bend knees and find your balance.

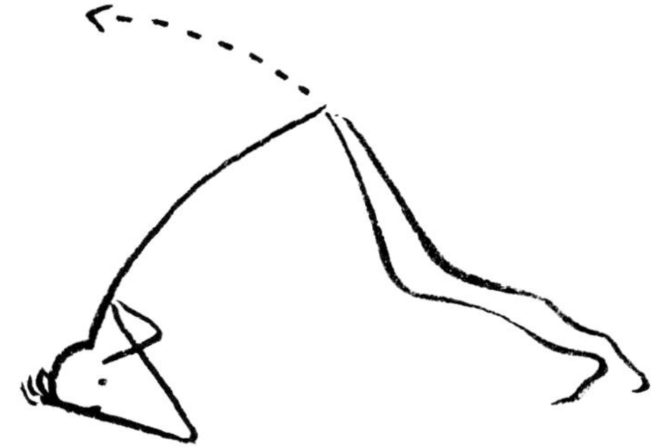

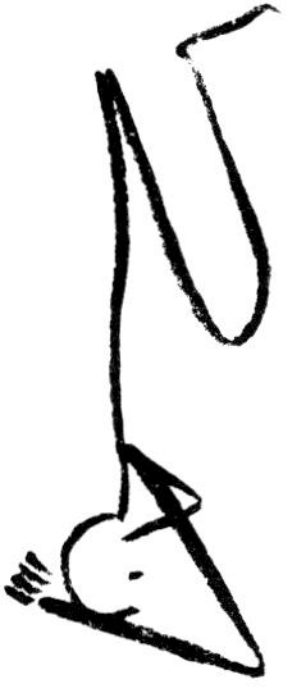

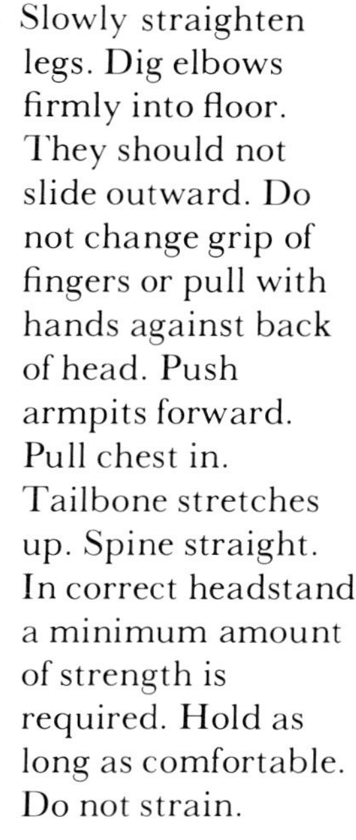

2. Slowly straighten legs. Dig elbows firmly into floor. They should not slide outward. Do not change grip of fingers or pull with hands against back of head. Push armpits forward. Pull chest in. Tailbone stretches up. Spine straight. In correct headstand a minimum amount of strength is required. Hold as long as comfortable. Do not strain.

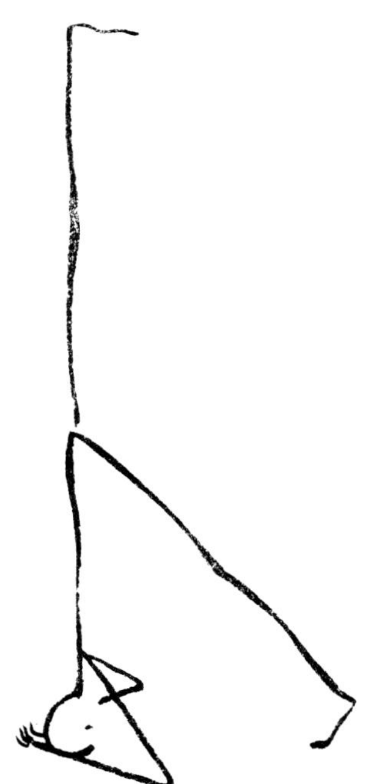

3. Move left foot down to touch floor. Bring leg back up, and repeat with other leg. Return to headstand position.

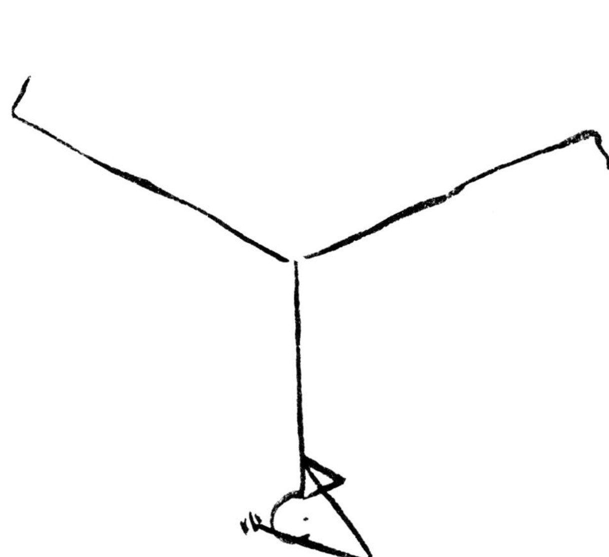

4. Then drop left leg forward and right leg backward. Repeat with other leg.

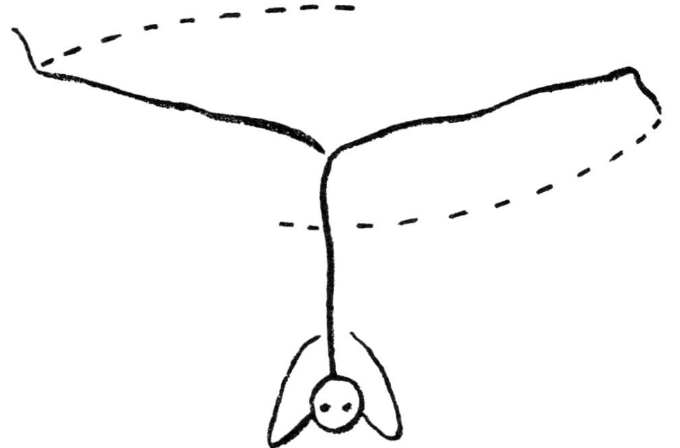

EXERCISE IX

1. From headstand position, twist trunk and turn pelvis to the left. Move right foot to the left, left foot to right. Hold. Bring legs back up straight and repeat on other side.

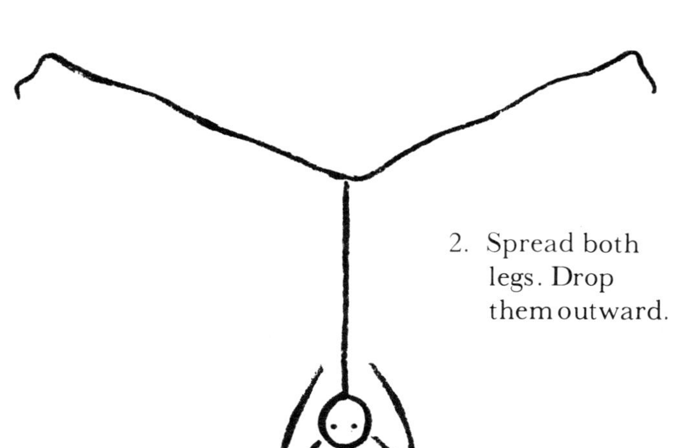

2. Spread both legs. Drop them outward.

3. Bend knees and bring soles of feet together. Push pelvis forward.

4. Falling out of headstand: Release hands and place them flat on floor. Tuck chin against chestbone and curve spine. Roll over and up.

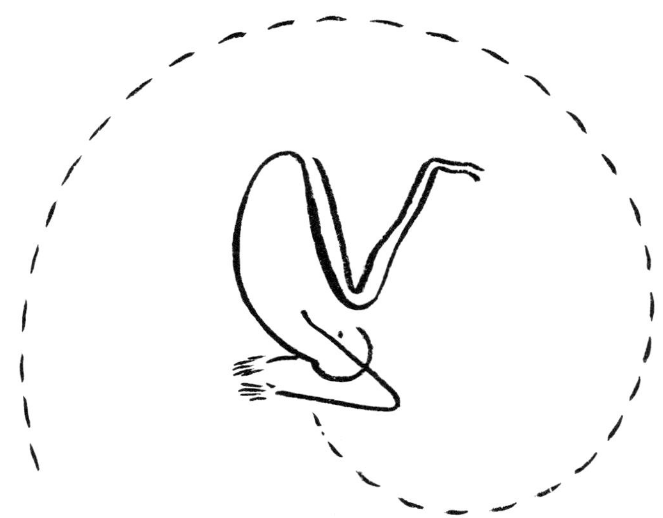

EXERCISE X

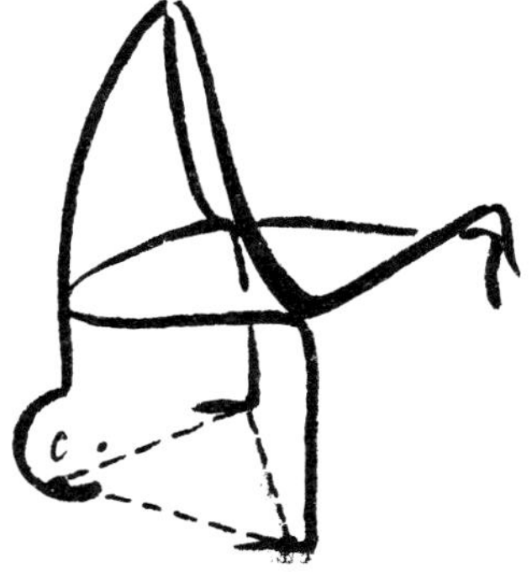

1. Crouch down. Place both hands on floor in line with shoulders. Hands form base of a triangle. Find a point on floor to complete triangle. Place top of head at this point. The triangle as a basis gives stability. Straighten spine, move buttocks upward and place knees on back of upper arms. Hold.

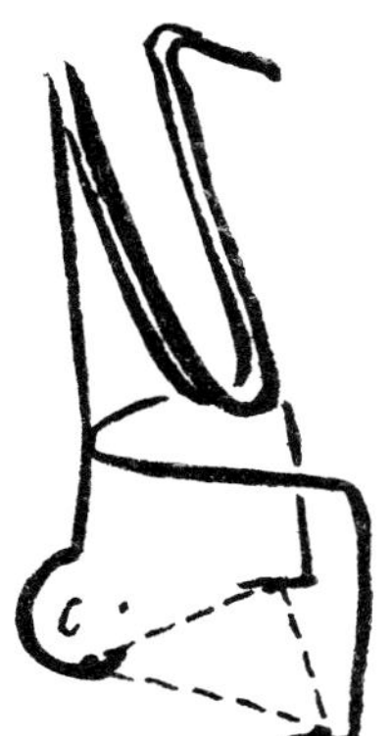

2. Straighten spine completely and lift knees off upper arms.

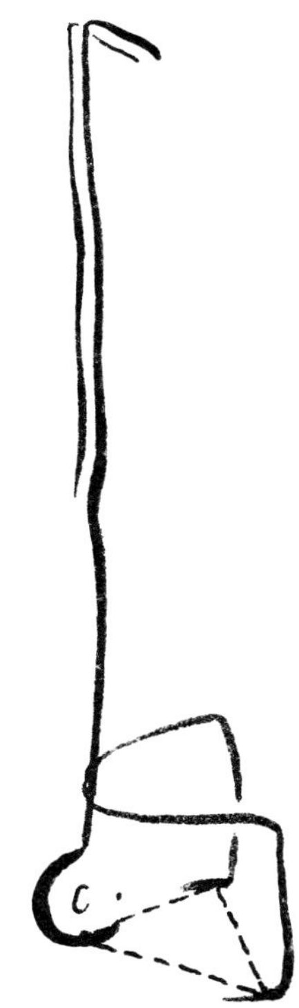

3. Straighten legs slowly. Hold. Come back down in reverse order. Repeat several times.

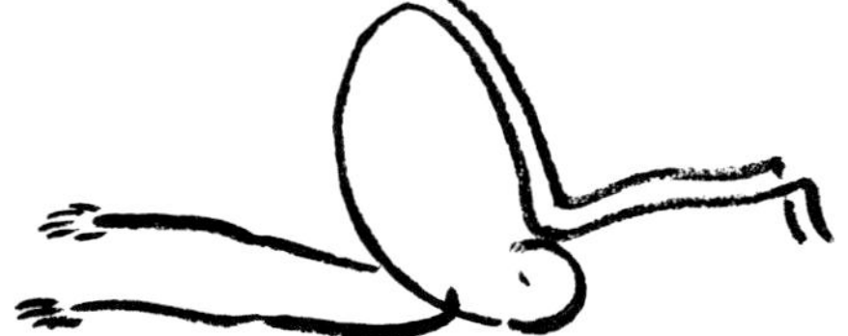

EXERCISE XI: SHOULDERSTAND

1. Lie on floor, legs and spine straight. Arms on floor next to body, palms down. Swing both legs over head and toward floor. Bend knees and rest them on forehead. Relax whole body and rest.

2. Straighten legs and place toes on floor. Push heels toward floor. Interlock fingers behind back and straighten arms. Shoulder blades pull together, shoulders move away from ears in direction of hands. Chestbone moves upward and toward face. Straighten spine; tailbone moves upward; hips move away from face.

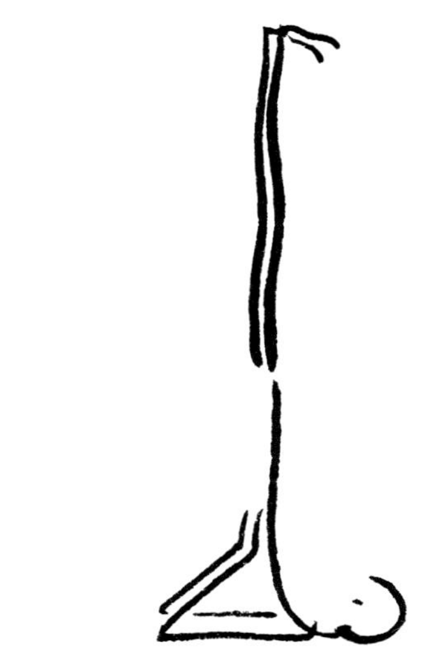

3. Keeping shoulders and elbows pulled together, release hands and place palms of hands on back, as near shoulders as possible. Then stretch both legs upward toward ceiling. Stretch heels upward, big toes together. Keep spine straight. Do not move your head in this position. Then return to starting position and lie down. Relax.

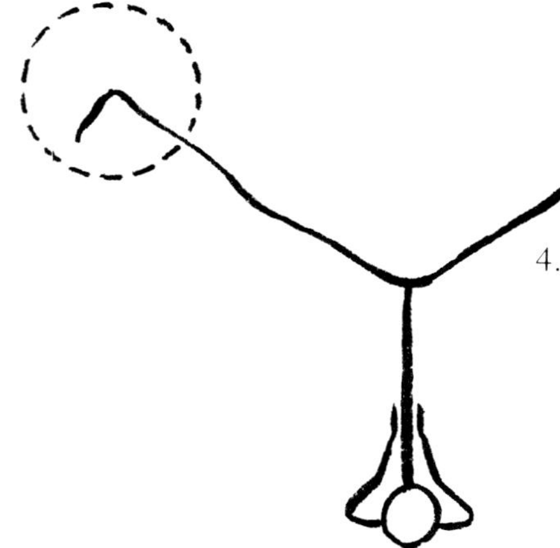

4. Return to shoulderstand position. Spread legs and drop them outward. Push pelvis forward. Turn ankles clockwise and anti-clockwise.

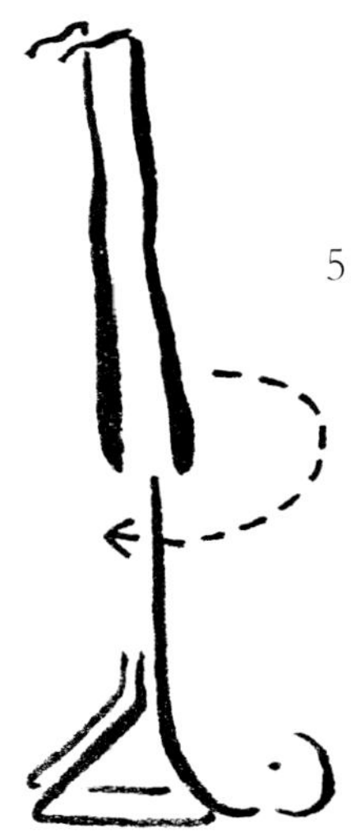

5. Stretch legs up again. While stretching, twist trunk and turn pelvis to face the right. Repeat on other side.

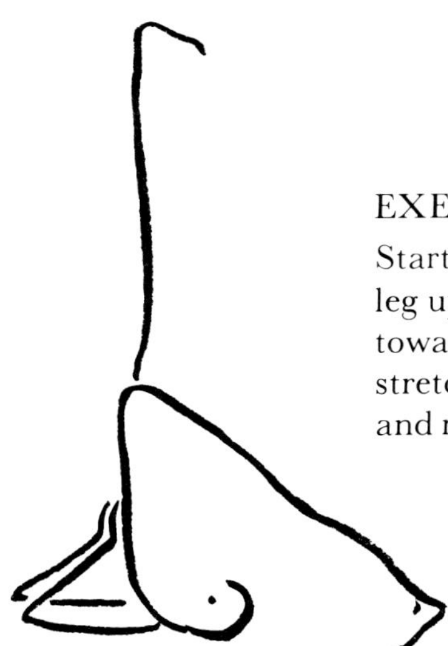

EXERCISE XII

Start in shoulderstand. Stretch left leg up while moving right foot down toward floor over head. Right heel stretches toward floor. Raise leg, and repeat on other side.

EXERCISE XIII

1. Start in shoulderstand. Bring both legs up straight. Bend knees, so that feet hang towards buttocks. Keep hipjoints straight.

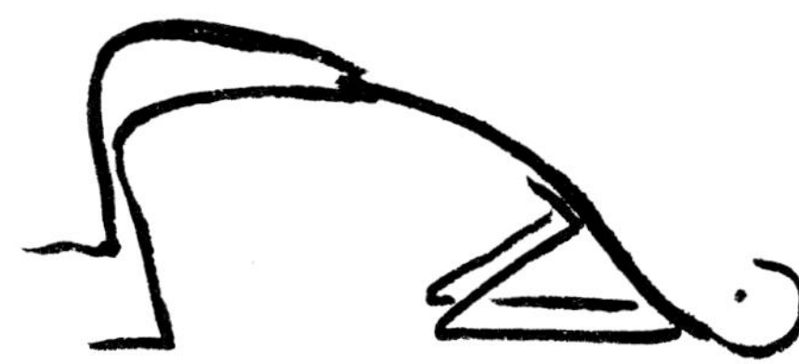

2. Then arch back and slowly bring both feet down flat on floor. Push pelvis upward.

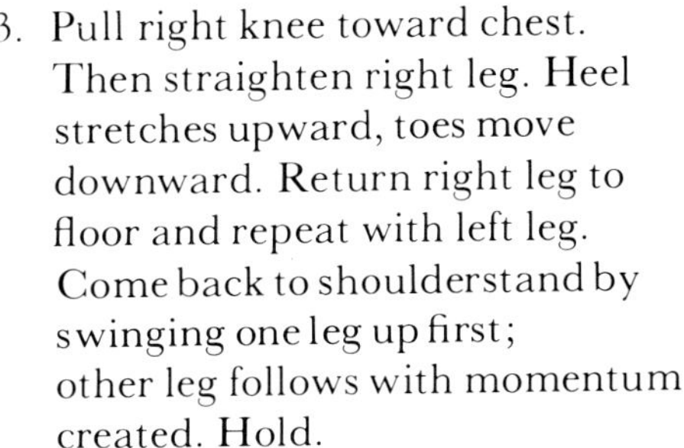

3. Pull right knee toward chest. Then straighten right leg. Heel stretches upward, toes move downward. Return right leg to floor and repeat with left leg. Come back to shoulderstand by swinging one leg up first; other leg follows with momentum created. Hold.

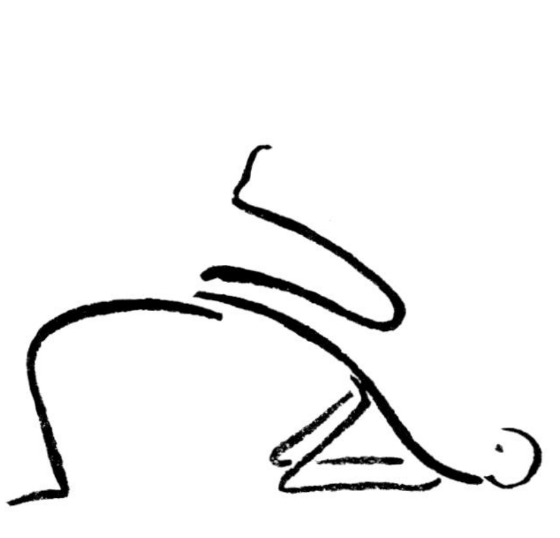

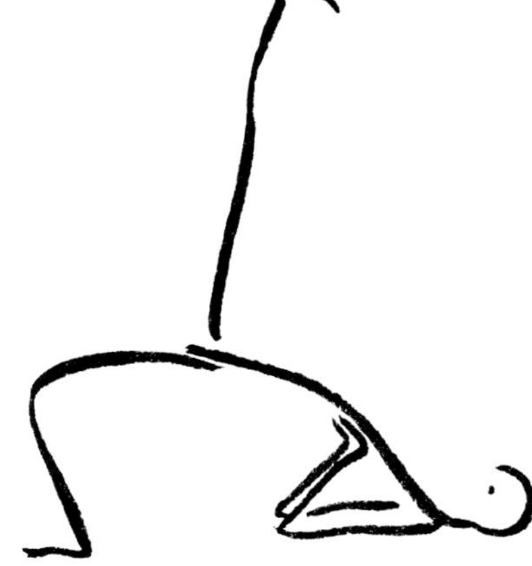

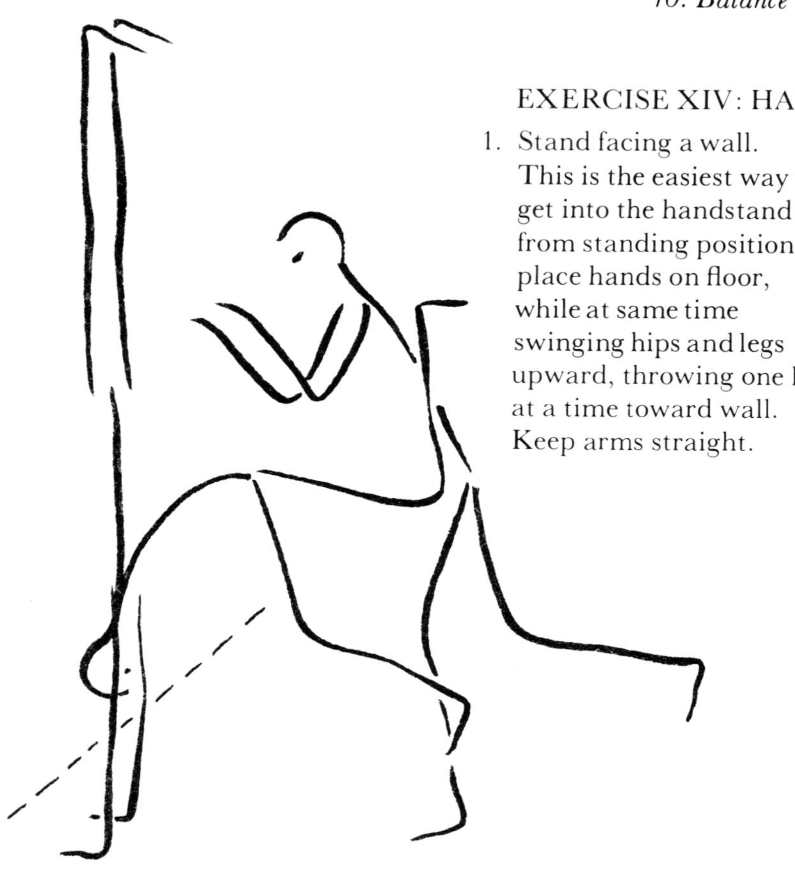

EXERCISE XIV: HANDSTAND

1. Stand facing a wall. This is the easiest way to get into the handstand: from standing position place hands on floor, while at same time swinging hips and legs upward, throwing one leg at a time toward wall. Keep arms straight.

2. When both feet contact wall, straighten legs and bring feet together. Straighten spine. Tailbone moves up. Pull chest in. Push shoulders away from wall, armpits forward. Take feet away from wall. Control balance by applying more or less pressure with fingertips into floor.

EXERCISE XV: ELBOWSTAND

Stand facing a wall. Place elbows on floor under shoulders, hands on floor in line with elbows. Palms face down, fingertips touch wall. Stand on toes and throw legs and hips upward and toward wall, one at a time. Rest feet together against wall, legs straight. Push shoulders away from wall, armpits forward. Head should not touch floor. Pull chest in. Straighten spine. Tailbone moves upward. Take feet away from wall. Balance is controlled by pressure of fingertips into floor.
When beginning this exercise, it may be helpful to tie a scarf around upper arms to prevent elbows from slipping outward and hands from sliding inward.

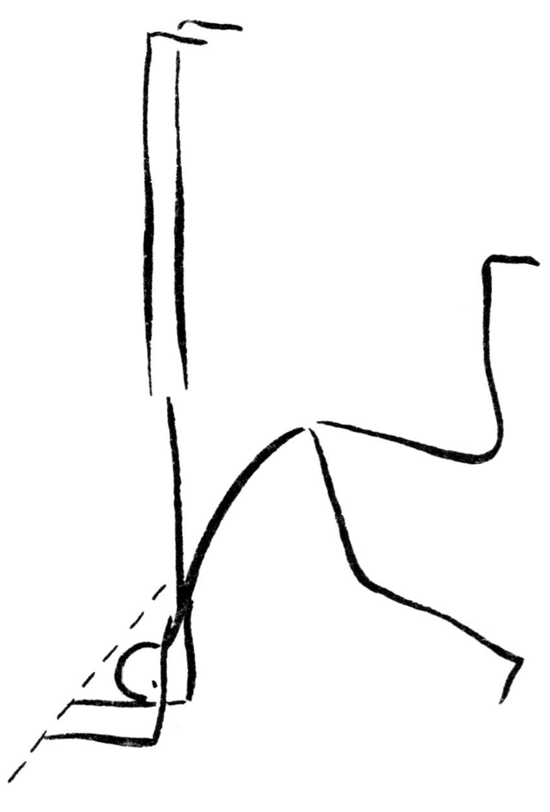

11. ENERGY

In order to know the feeling of energy in its increasing forms, the increase must be reached with a further extension of energy in a formerly unused area. A muscle is composed of thousands of muscle fibres. The muscle fibre is either in use or unused. There is no middle ground. When you get to a certain point, it is ON. Until you get there, it is OFF. Flow is the way to get there: like waves coming in at high tide, always further and further in, each time with a sliding slipping back, but on again still further to fulfil the potential of the body. This chapter is planned as a sequence of exercises but you can also do them separately or in another order.

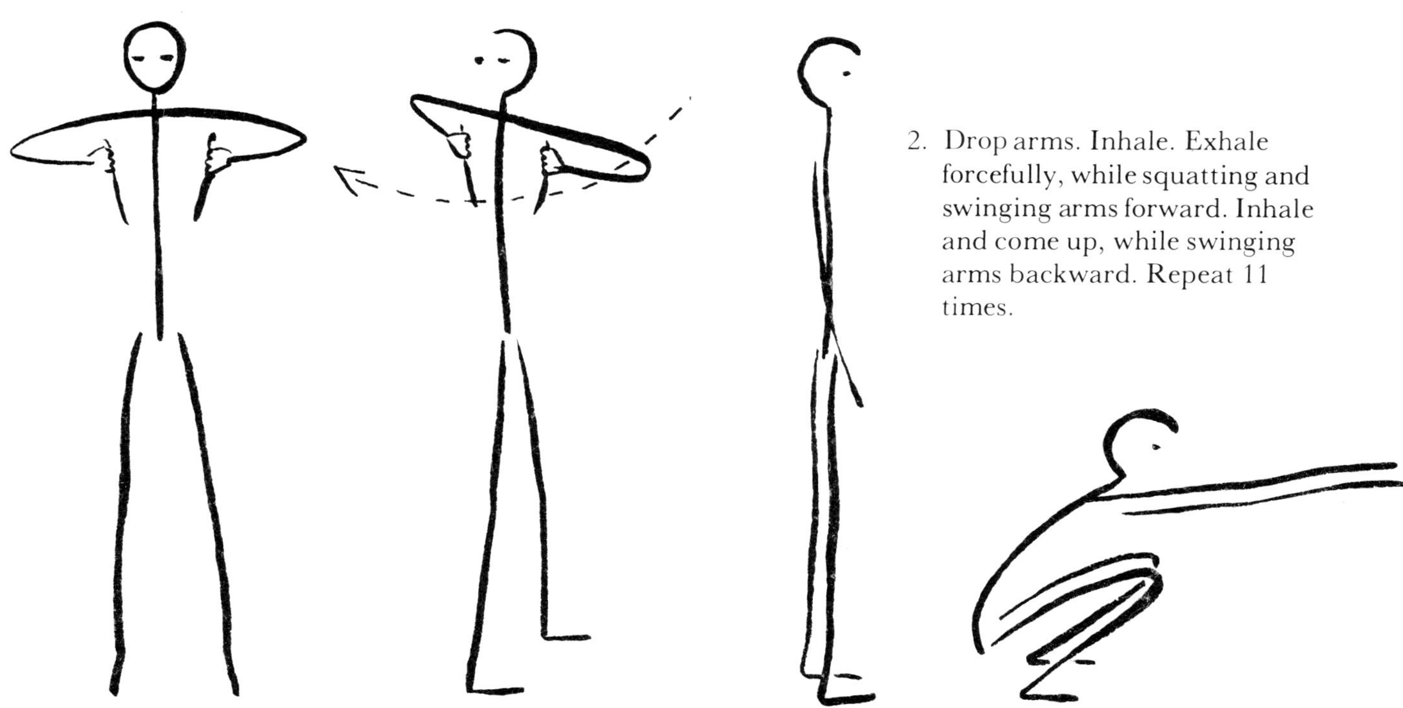

2. Drop arms. Inhale. Exhale forcefully, while squatting and swinging arms forward. Inhale and come up, while swinging arms backward. Repeat 11 times.

1. Stand with feet one foot apart. Place fists in side of ribs and inhale. Then exhale forcefully while turning shoulders and trunk to right. Look over right shoulder at wall behind you. Inhale, while returning to starting position. Then exhale forcefully, while turning to left. Twist from right to left and back. Repeat 22 times.

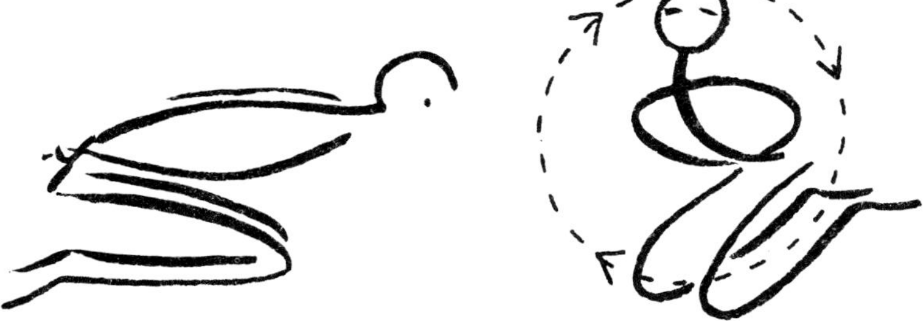

3. Kneel down. Bring arms behind back, right hand holds left wrist. Lean trunk forward. Drop head. Bring head up over right shoulder in a circular movement, while inhaling through nose. Exhale forcefully through mouth, and drop head down in a circular movement over left shoulder.

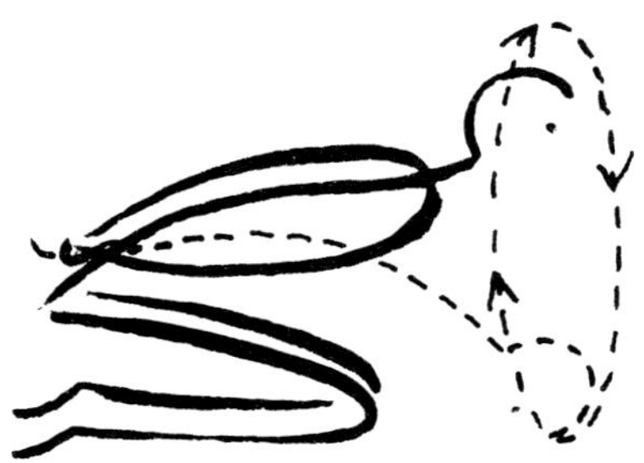

4. By turning trunk you can swing your head round in a circular movement, while keeping neck relaxed. The head swings around like a ball on a string. Exhale each time head swings downward. Repeat 22 times.

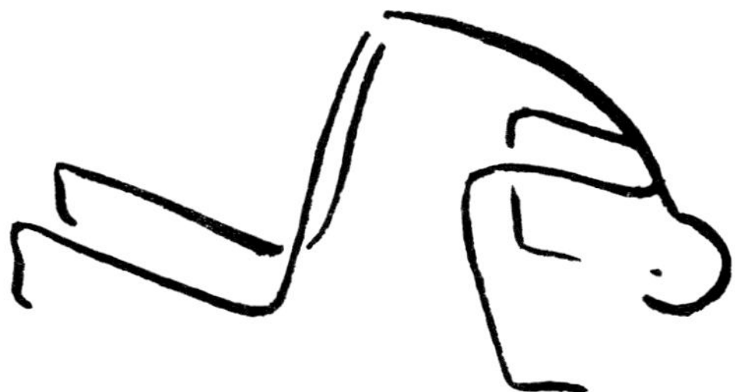

5. Place top of head and palms on floor, or else do a headstand. Keep knees apart. Inhale deeply and slowly through nose in five counts, then exhale forcefully through mouth in five counts, as if blowing out a candle behind you. Repeat 11 times.

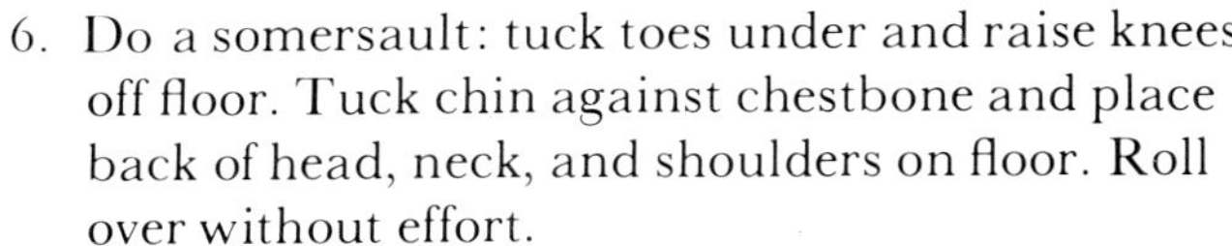

6. Do a somersault: tuck toes under and raise knees off floor. Tuck chin against chestbone and place back of head, neck, and shoulders on floor. Roll over without effort.

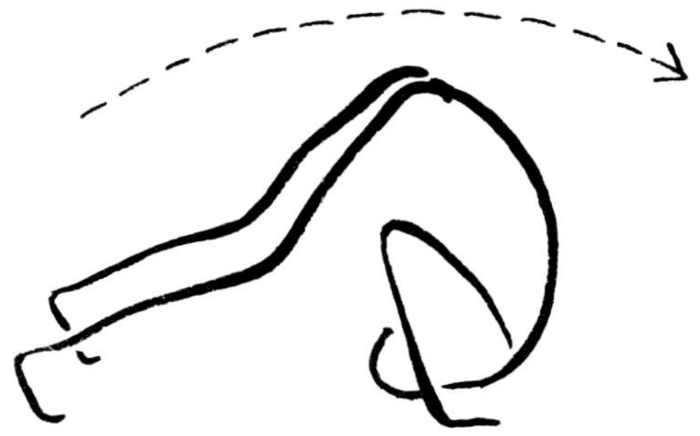

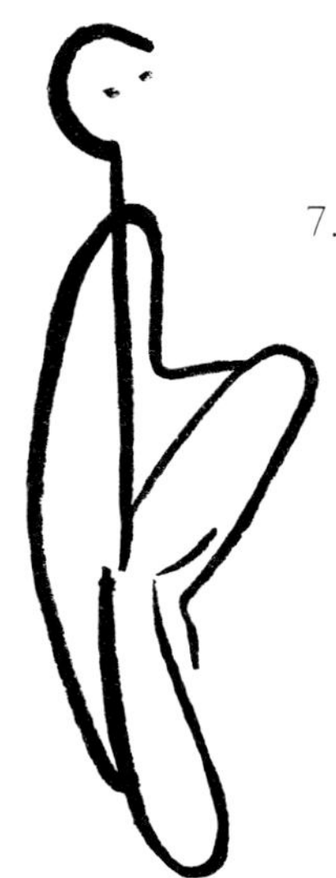

7. From somersault sit up into easy position. Straighten spine. Hands under knees. Inhale slowly and deeply through nose in five counts.

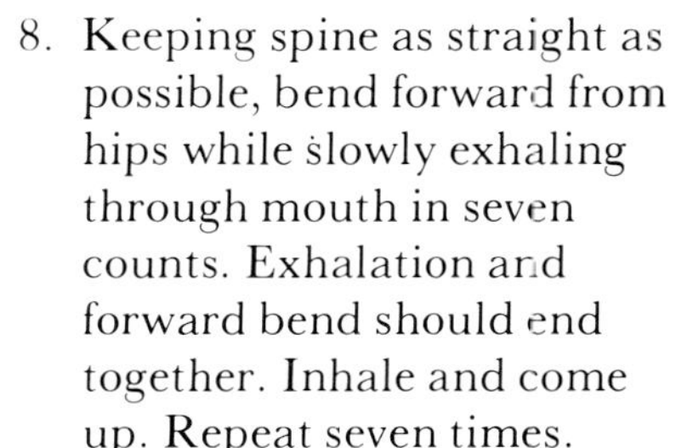

8. Keeping spine as straight as possible, bend forward from hips while slowly exhaling through mouth in seven counts. Exhalation and forward bend should end together. Inhale and come up. Repeat seven times.

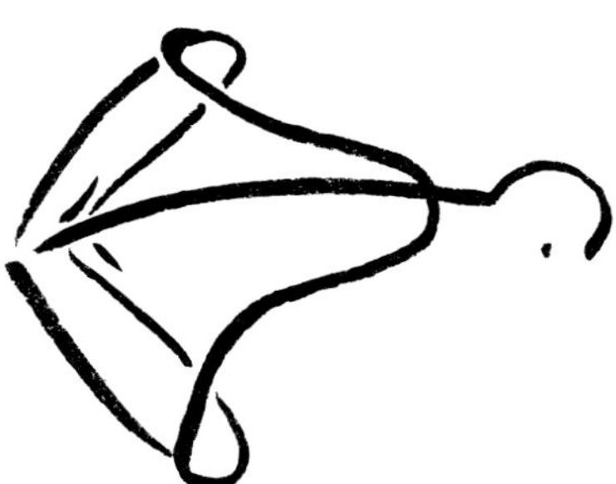

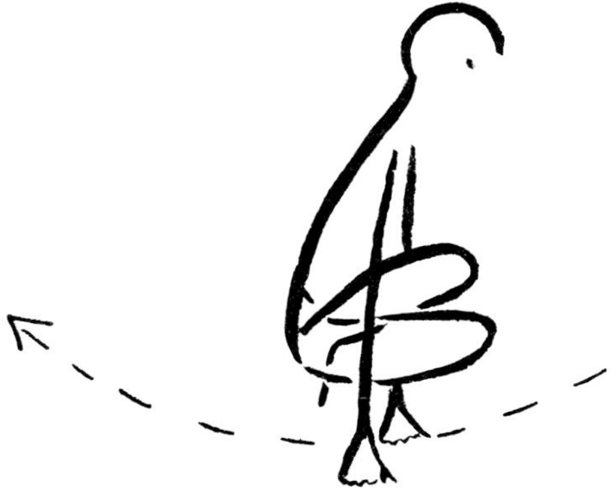

9. Still sitting in the easy position, place both hands, fists, or fingertips on floor next to hips. Lift body up on hands; buttocks and legs come off the floor.

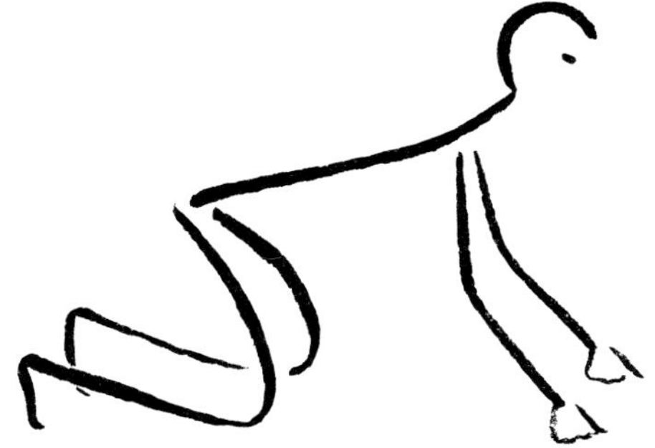

10. Then swing both legs backward between arms and end up kneeling on all fours.

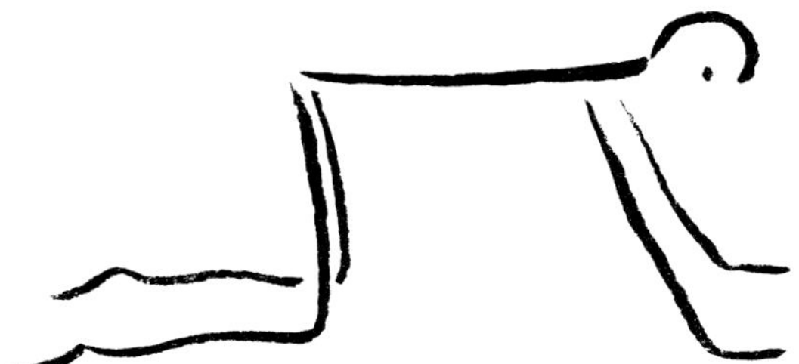

11. Then move hands about two feet in front of knees, palms down. Tops of feet touch floor. Inhale deeply through nose. Hold. Dig hands firmly into floor and at the same time slowly pull hips backward. Spine, sides of chest, and armpits will stretch.
This is a dual movement; hands press down and forward while back stretches backward and down.

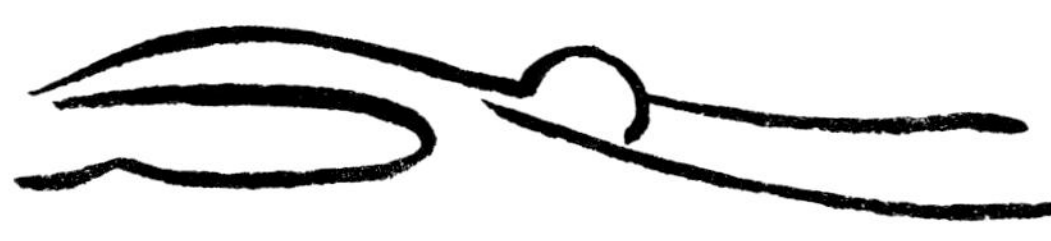

12. When buttocks touch heels and chest touches knees, exhale in an explosive way. Then relax.
Inhale through nose, hold breath and come back up. Exhale. Repeat this movement 11 times.

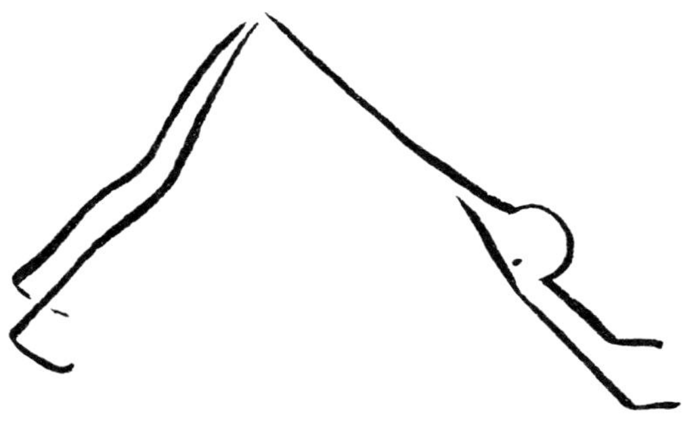

13. From kneeling position come up to stand on hands and toes. Take a deep breath through nose and hold.

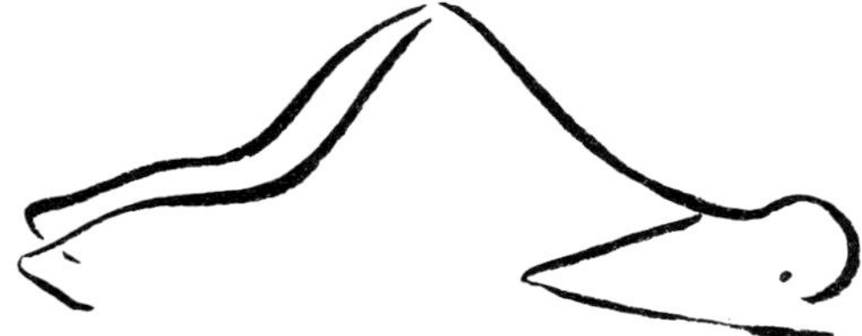

14. While holding breath, bend elbows and move face downward until nose touches floor between hands.

15. Move nose forward over floor until body is straight and stomach contacts floor.

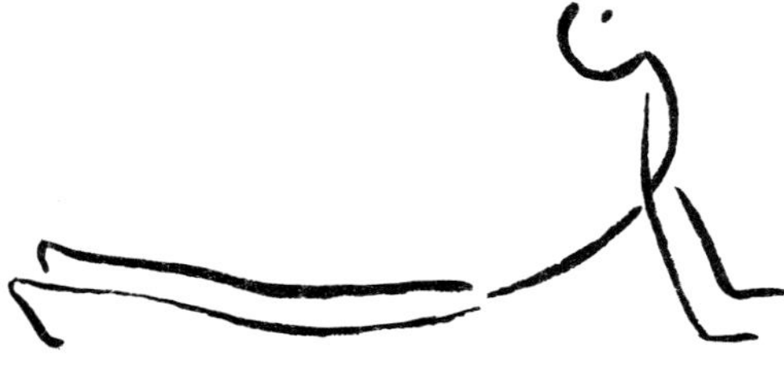

16. Still holding breath, straighten arms, arch spine, and look up. Drop head backward.

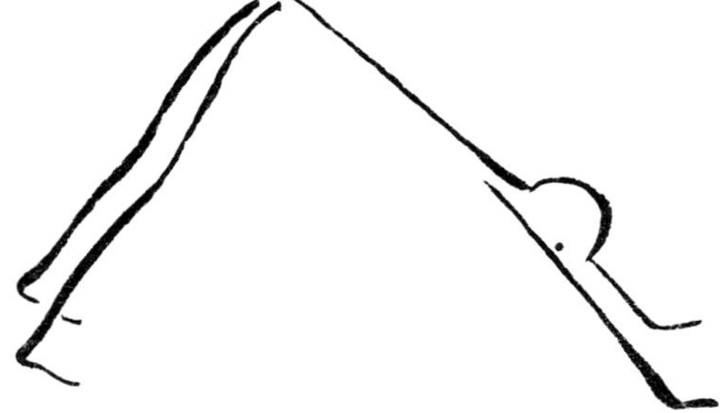

17. Reverse movement of hips and come standing on hands and toes again, exhaling forcefully through mouth. Repeat this cycle 7 times.

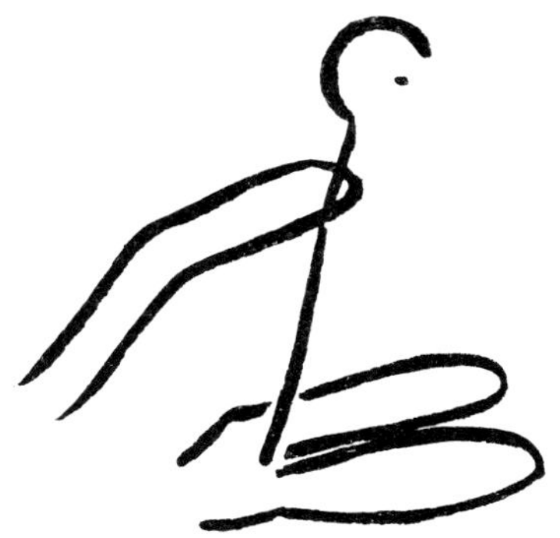

18. From last position put knees on floor and sit down between feet. Feet curl around buttocks, tops of feet on floor and buttocks on floor. (Or sit on heels.)

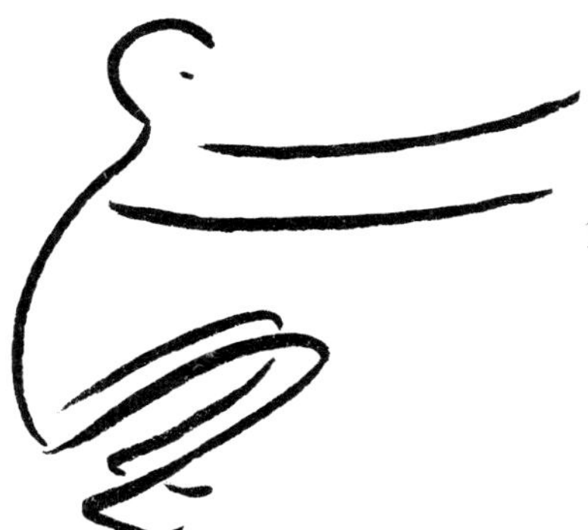

19. Then jump up into crouching position without touching floor with hands.

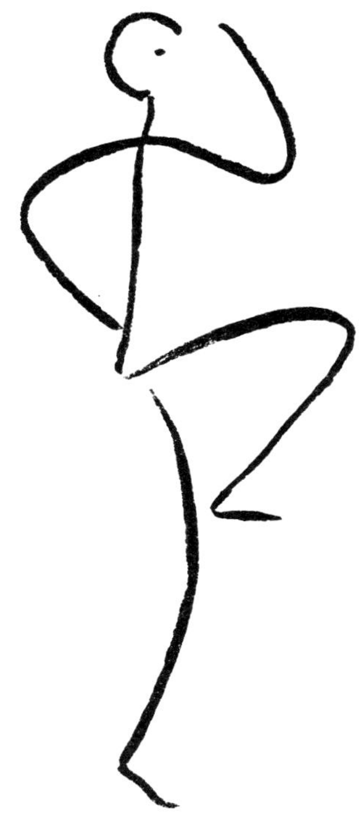

20. Now stand up and start running on the spot. Exhale through mouth every fourth step. Pull knees up high. Maintain for at least 100 steps.

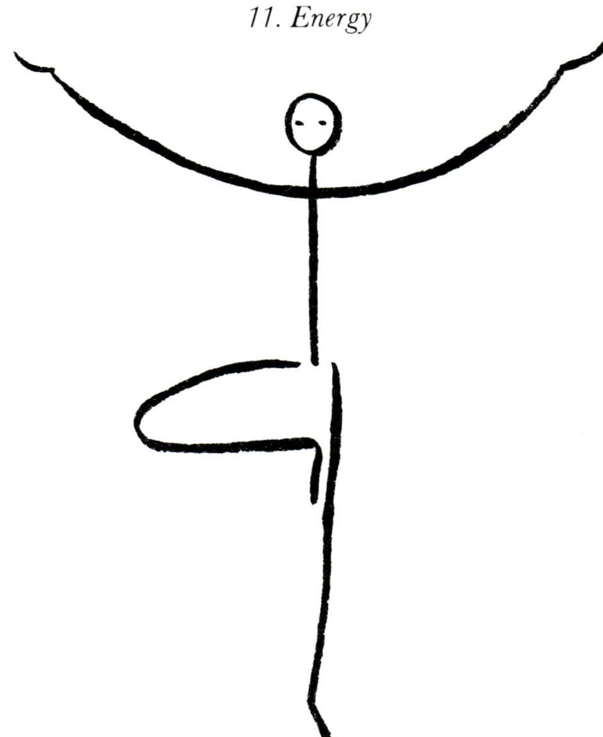

21. After jogging, place right foot on inside of left thigh. Spread arms out, hands reaching upward, palms up. Breathe rhythmically, holding each inhalation and exhalation five counts. Repeat each step five times.

In through nose. Out through nose.
In through nose. Out through mouth.
In through mouth. Out through nose.
In through mouth. Out through mouth.
In through nose. Hold five counts.
Out through nose.

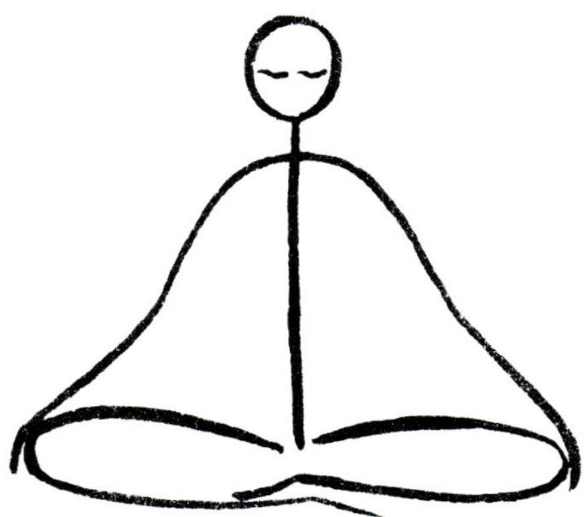

22. Sit in easy position. Relax completely and breathe as silently and lightly as possible. Continue for ten minutes.

12. RELAXATION

When you are relaxed there should be no voluntary effort of the muscles. Imagine you have just died, and your body is lying on its back in the corpse position, pulled against the earth by gravity. The more you can relax, the more your body will be in contact with the floor. Feel how your body contacts the floor today. Move your awareness to the tailbone. Without moving, feel the tailbone. In your mind wiggle your tailbone from right to left. As a foetus you used to have a tail; some of that feeling must still be there. So, wag your tail. When this feeling has become quite clear and pleasant, move one vertebra upwards. In your imagination try to move it from right to left. When the contact is clear, move up to the next vertebra. Continue upward, mentally wiggling each vertebra in the spine until you reach the base of the skull. Then reverse the process, so that your energy moves back down to the tailbone, vertebra by vertebra.

It will be more difficult to feel each of the fused vertebrae; but at least you can feel the tailbone, points in the sacrum, and each of the 24 vertebrae that are capable of movement. In the beginning this may seem impossible. As your awareness grows, and you get more in contact with your feelings, you will be able to feel each vertebra separately. When your spine is no longer a mystery to you, you will be able to heal any kind of discomfort in the spine.

Now lie on the floor with your feet about two feet apart, hands away from the body. Check that the weight of the body is equally distributed over the right and left sides. Lift your head and look at your feet and hips to check that they are symmetrical. When you lower your head, do so with a slightly tucked-in chin, stretching your neck a bit. Avoid arching the neck. Relax body, close your eyes. Move your awareness to the back of your heels and feel how they touch the floor. Move slowly up into the ankles; then calves, knees, thighs, buttocks, lower back, middle part of the back, upper part of the back. Feel how the shoulders contact the floor; then the upper arms, elbows, lower arms, wrists, hands. Your skeleton is made in such a way that, in a perfectly relaxed position, the whole of the skeleton can sink into the floor.

Continue lying on the floor. Relax. Eyes are closed. Feel your body as it contacts the floor. Then let go and move your awareness to the right foot – nothing but that right foot. Without moving it, feel it completely. Try to feel the footbones, each individual toe, the ball of the foot, the hollow of the foot, the heel, the back of the foot. Feel the warmth of the foot inside. (If you learn to relax and concentrate properly, you will be able to affect your body temperature.) Then move your awareness to the right ankle: nothing but that ankle. Try to feel the skin on the outside and the inside. Feel the warmth inside the ankle. Follow this warm glow slowly upward into the lower leg. Feel the calf muscle touching the floor, feel the shin, feel the blood in the veins and arteries, feel the bones, feel the warmth moving upward. Then move your awareness to your knee. Try to feel inside the knee joint, how it is constructed. Feel the knee cap and the warmth inside it. Move upwards into the thigh. Feel the whole length of the thigh bone. Try to feel the different muscles, the blood running through the veins, the separate cells inside, and always the warmth. Now concentrate on the whole of the leg. Feel how it has changed by your concentration. Its temperature should now be higher than the other leg's.

Move your awareness to the left hand. Try to forget everything but that left hand. There is a tremendous concentration of muscles and nerves in the hands (and feet and face), so it is easy to feel every part of the hand. Feel the fingertips, each finger separately, the nails, the top of the hand, the lines in your hand, the bones in your hand, the inside of your hand. Feel how the arteries send blood to the fingertips and the veins carry it back to the heart. Feel the warmth inside. Then let go and move your awareness to your wrist. Feel the wristbones and your pulse. If you lie still, it is very easy to feel your pulse without touching the wrist with your right hand. Now move to the lower arm. Feel the part of the arm that touches the floor. Feel the skin, the blood inside the capillaries, the armbones, and the warmth inside. Let go of the lower arm and concentrate on the elbow: only the elbow. Then move into the upper arm. Feel inside, feel the bone, the skin, the different muscles, the warm glow filling the entire arm with a pleasant feeling. Let the arm get heavier and heavier. Then move into the shoulder and take your time to feel it. Relax it inside. Then let go and once more move your awareness to the whole arm and feel how it has changed by your concentration.

Now move your awareness to a point slightly above the navel. In many disciplines this extremely sensitive spot, known as the 'solar plexus', is considered as the centre of the body: 'ki' in karate, 'hara' in Buddhism, 'fire chakra' in yogic discipline. Rest right hand on stomach, slightly above the navel, and concentrate on the warmth that you feel inside. Let the warmth swell a bit and then sink toward floor into your spine. When the glow has reached your spine and you can really feel it, hold it. You can stop here. Let your mind drift and start to dream half-consciously. Imagine yourself lying in a wonderful forest. You are lying on warm sand. The sun is shining. It is close to evening. The birds have begun to sing again. The flowers give off an enchanting fragrance. Smell it. The centre of your body feels safe and warm and strong. There seems to be no time. No other human being is around or seems to have ever been here. You look at the sky. There are some clouds. They take on definite shapes. One looks like a dog, another like your mother. You hear the leaves rustle in the bushes. A deer and its young have appeared and come to smell your body.

When you decide to return to tangible reality, to leave your creation, realise that the kind of life you lead has been created by you and your thoughts, consciously or unconsciously. Our lives are our thoughts; we create the world inside. We are responsible for our bodies and our feelings. As we become more aware, as we feel our energy level flowing and growing, we can even begin to change and re-create the world outside us. Imagination will become reality.